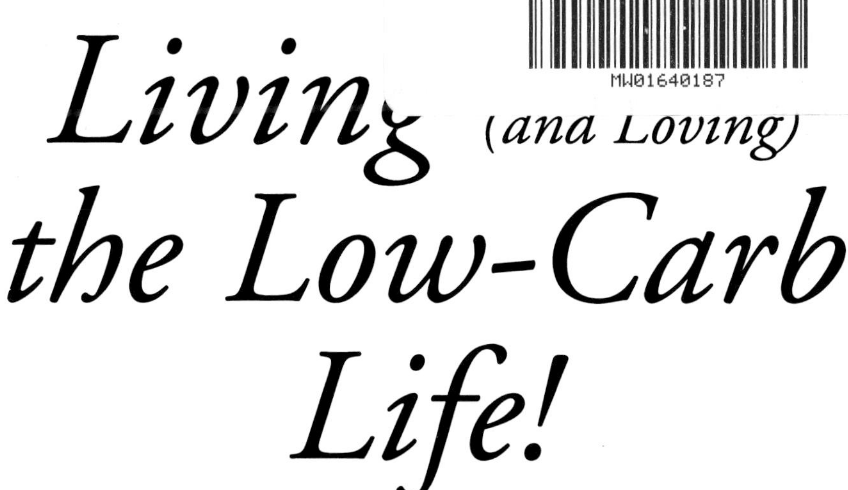

DARLIN
Publications

Printed in the United States of America

Recipe photographs on front cover:
Bacon & Onion Omelet (Page 18)
Lasagna (page 48)
Pumpkin Pie (Page 153)

If you have any questions or comments concerning this book, please write:

Darlin Publications
P.O. Box 7178
The Woodlands, TX 77378

Contents

Contents

Contents

Contents

Contents

Contents

Appetizers & Snacks

Taco Dip

Makes 10 servings.

12 ounces cream cheese softened
1/2 cup sour cream
2 teaspoons chili powder
1 1/2 teaspoons ground cumin
1/8 teaspoon ground red pepper
1/2 cup Picante sauce
lettuce leaves
1 cup Cheddar cheese shredded
1 cup Monterey jack cheese shredded
1/2 cup plum tomatoes diced
1/3 cup green onions sliced
Pork skins

Combine cream cheese, sour cream, chili powder, cumin and red pepper in large bowl. Mix well until blended. Stir in salsa. Spread dip onto lettuce-lined service platter. Top with Cheddar cheese and Monterey Jack cheese, tomatoes and green onions. Serve with pork skins.

Per serving (excluding unknown items): 241.4 Calories; 21.9 Fat (79.8 calories from fat); 8.9 Protein; 3.6 Carbohydrate; 64 Cholesterol; 331 Sodium.

Chicken Salad Balls

Makes 12 servings.

1 cup chicken cooked and chopped
1 tablespoon onion chopped
2 tablespoons pimiento chopped
dash hot sauce
salt and pepper
1/2 cup mayonnaise-type salad dressing
1/2 cup pecans chopped

Combine and mix well all ingredients. Chill for three to four hours. Shape into 1-inch balls. Yields: 2 dozen.

Per serving (excluding unknown items): 79.9 Calories; 5.9 Fat (65.7 calories from fat); 3.8 Protein; 3.1 Carbohydrate; 13 Cholesterol; 80 Sodium.

Pimento Cheese Spread

Makes 10 servings.

12 ounces American cheese diced
2 teaspoons Worcestershire sauce
10 tablespoons mayonnaise
1/2 packet Sweet 'n Low® sweetener
1 teaspoon garlic powder
1 teaspoon onion powder

Mix all ingredients. Serving size is two tablespoons.

Per serving (excluding unknown items): 229.0 Calories; 22.3 Fat (84.9 calories from fat); 7.8 Protein; 1.1 Carbohydrate; 37 Cholesterol; 309 Sodium.

Tuna Devil Eggs

Makes 8 servings.

1 1/2 dozen eggs hard boiled
1 can tuna in water
dash salt and pepper
3 tablespoons mayonnaise-type salad dressing
2 teaspoons mustard
1/2 onion chopped

Boil eggs with a little salt. Cut eggs in half and take out the yolks. Mash yolks with a fork, adding salt, pepper, salad dressing, tuna, mustard and chopped onion. Fill egg whites with the mixture.

Per serving (excluding unknown items): 61.4 Calories; 2.9 Fat (42.7 calories from fat); 6.4 Protein; 2.3 Carbohydrate; 42 Cholesterol; 134 Sodium.

Cheesy Sausage Balls

Makes 4 servings.

1 pound pork sausage
12 ounces cheddar cheese grated
1/4 cup soy flour

Preheat oven to 325 degrees. Mix ingredients and roll into 16 small balls. Place on baking sheet and bake until done (approximately 15 minutes). Each sausage ball is approximately one gram of carbohyrate.

Per serving (excluding unknown items): 838.8 Calories; 75.0 Fat (80.7 calories from fat); 36.3 Protein; 4.1 Carbohydrate; 166 Cholesterol; 1285 Sodium.

Fried Cheese

Makes 1 serving.

4 ounces mozzarella cheese cut in 1/4" strips
2 eggs slightly beaten
1/2 cup pork skins crushed

Dip cheese sticks into eggs. Roll in finely crushed pork skins. Fry in 1/2-inch deep oil on medium heat until browned on all sides.
NOTE: To keep cheese from melting during frying, keep very cold in the refrigerator.

Per serving (excluding unknown items): 599.0 Calories; 43.4 Fat (66.1 calories from fat); 46.2 Protein; 3.8 Carbohydrate; 496 Cholesterol; 1037 Sodium.

Guacamole Dip

Makes 8 servings.

1 cup cottage cheese
1 medium avocado cut in chunks
1 tomato cut in chunks
2 tablespoons lemon juice
1 tablespoon Worcestershire sauce
1 teaspoon garlic salt
1/8 teaspoon cayenne pepper

Combine cottage cheese, avocado, tomato, lemon juice, Worcestershire, garlic salt and cayenne in blender. Blend until smooth. Serve as a dip with fresh vegetables or pork skins. Makes about two cups.

Per serving (excluding unknown items): 58.3 Calories; 3.4 Fat (50.4 calories from fat); 4.3 Protein; 3.2 Carbohydrate; 2 Cholesterol; 391 Sodium.

Chili Con Queso

Makes 12 servings.

3 tablespoons oil
1/2 cup onion chopped
1 clove garlic minced
1 teaspoon chili powder
14 ounces tomatoes, canned drained and chopped
1/2 packet Sweet 'n Low® sweetener
4 ounces green chiles drained and chopped
4 ounces cheddar cheese grated
4 ounces Monterey jack cheese grated

Place in a skillet the oil, onion, garlic and chili powder. Saute until onion is tender-crisp. Add tomatoes, sweetener and chilies. Bring to a boil. Add both cheeses. Heat until cheeses are melted. Serve with Pork Skins or pour over scrambled eggs.

Per serving (excluding unknown items): 116.5 Calories; 9.6 Fat (72.6 calories from fat); 5.2 Protein; 2.9 Carbohydrate; 18 Cholesterol; 166 Sodium.

Country Ham-Stuffed Eggs

Makes 2 servings.

3 hard-boiled eggs
1/3 cup ham finely chopped
1/8 teaspoon dry mustard
2 tablespoons mayonnaise

Cut the eggs in half lengthwise and carefully scoop out the yolks into a mixing bowl. Add the remaining ingredients to the yolks and mash with a fork until the mixture is well blended. Mound the yolk mixture into the whites and sprinkle the yolk mixture lightly with paprika.

Per serving (excluding unknown items): 240.3 Calories; 20.9 Fat (77.4 calories from fat); 12.3 Protein; 1.5 Carbohydrate; 288 Cholesterol; 464 Sodium.

Ham Pinwheels

Makes 1 serving.

4 ham slices
cream cheese whipped

Spread thin ham slices with whipped cream cheese. Roll up and chill. Cut into 1-1/4 inch pieces.

Per serving (excluding unknown items): 192.4 Calories; 14.5 Fat (69.3 calories from fat); 14.4 Protein; 0.0 Carbohydrate; 43 Cholesterol; 1152 Sodium.

Jalapeno Cheese Squares

Makes 8 servings.

4 eggs beaten
1 teaspoon onion minced
1 can green chiles minced
4 cups cheddar cheese shredded

Preheat oven to 350 degrees. Mix all ingredients well. Spread into ungreased 8-inch square pan. Bake for 30 minutes.

Per serving (excluding unknown items): 261.7 Calories; 20.9 Fat (72.2 calories from fat); 16.9 Protein; 1.3 Carbohydrate; 151 Cholesterol; 379 Sodium.

Avocado Dip

Makes 8 servings.

2 avocados mashed
2 teaspoons grated onion
1 lemon juiced
salt to taste
1 chili pepper diced
1 tablespoon mayonnaise

Mix all ingredients well. Chill. Serve with pork skins or vegetable sticks.

Per serving (excluding unknown items): 76.8 Calories; 7.2 Fat (74.2 calories from fat); 1.0 Protein; 4.6 Carbohydrate; 1 Cholesterol; 14 Sodium.

Deviled Eggs

Makes 6 servings.

6 eggs
3 tablespoons mayonnaise
1 teaspoon mustard
1/4 teaspoon pepper
1/8 teaspoon salt
1 teaspoon sweet pickle relish

Hard boil the eggs and peel. Cut peeled eggs lengthwise into halves. Slip out yolks; mash with fork. Mix in mayonnaise, mustard, pepper and salt. Stir in sweet pickle relish. Fill whites with egg yolk mixture, heaping it lightly.

Per serving (excluding unknown items): 114.6 Calories; 10.1 Fat (78.2 calories from fat); 5.4 Protein; 0.9 Carbohydrate; 186 Cholesterol; 154 Sodium.

Crab Ball Hors d'Oeuvre

Makes 4 servings.

1 cup crab meat
8 ounces cream cheese softened
2 teaspoons chives chopped
1/4 teaspoon garlic powder
1/4 teaspoon salt
1/2 cup pecans chopped

Thaw and drain crab meat. Blend softened cream cheese, chives, garlic powder and salt. Fold in crab meat. Shape into log or ball. Roll in pecans. Serve with fresh vegetables.

Per serving (excluding unknown items): 279.8 Calories; 25.0 Fat (79.2 calories from fat); 11.8 Protein; 3.0 Carbohydrate; 92 Cholesterol; 413 Sodium.

Breakfast & Brunch

Huevos Rancheros

Makes 4 servings.

3 tablespoons butter
2 tablespoons onion finely chopped
1 clove garlic minced
2 tablespoons green pepper finely chopped
6 eggs
2 tablespoons picante sauce

Melt butter in large frying pan. Saute onions, garlic, and pepper until soft. Beat eggs until light and pour into frying pan. Cook over very low heat, stirring constantly. When eggs begin to harden, add picante sauce, continuing to cook and stir until eggs are set. Serve immediately.

Per serving (excluding unknown items): 176.1 Calories; 15.0 Fat (76.7 calories from fat); 8.2 Protein; 2.1 Carbohydrate; 298 Cholesterol; 222 Sodium.

Cheese-Baked Eggs

Makes 2 servings.

2 eggs
2 tablespoons cheddar cheese grated
2 tablespoons butter
2 tablespoons heavy cream
salt
pepper

Preheat oven to 375 degrees. Fill a baking dish halfway with water and heat to a simmer. Divide one teaspoon of butter into the bottom of two custard cups. Divide one tablespoon of cheese into each cup. Carefully break an egg into each cup. Place one tablespoon of cream over each egg. Top with remaining cheese. Place cups in baking dish and place in the oven. Bake for 10 minutes. Salt and pepper to taste.

Per serving (excluding unknown items): 243.5 Calories; 23.5 Fat (86.1 calories from fat); 7.5 Protein; 1.0 Carbohydrate; 242 Cholesterol; 219 Sodium.

Sausage Casserole

Makes 10 servings.

2 pounds pork sausage patties
1 can chili peppers chopped
1 pound monterey jack cheese grated
8 eggs
salt and pepper

Fry sausage, drain and place in casserole dish. Spread chili peppers over sausage. Spread cheese over sausage/chili mixture. (Cover and refrigerate or freeze.) When ready to serve, beat eggs mixed with salt and pepper. Pour over top. Bake at 350 degrees for 45 minutes.

Per serving (excluding unknown items): 600.1 Calories; 53.8 Fat (81.2 calories from fat); 26.0 Protein; 2.0 Carbohydrate; 249 Cholesterol; 1460 Sodium.

Bacon and Onion Omelet

Makes 1 serving.

2 eggs
splash heavy cream
2 tablespoons butter
2 tablespoons onion chopped
2 slices bacon crumbled
1/2 cup American cheese shredded

Saute onions in butter in a frying pan. Cook and crumble the bacon. Set onions and bacon aside. Add a splash of cream to eggs and beat. Pour into frying pan. Sprinkle eggs with crumbled bacon, sauted onions and cheese. When firm, fold in half. Flip egg over. Cook until done.

Per serving (excluding unknown items): 620.8 Calories; 55.2 Fat (79.9 calories from fat); 27.5 Protein; 3.7 Carbohydrate; 492 Cholesterol; 910 Sodium.

One-Skillet Breakfast

Makes 4 servings.

6 slices bacon
1 tomato diced
1/2 cup cheddar cheese grated
6 eggs beaten
salt and pepper

Cook bacon and drain. Add to hot fat and cook about three minutes the diced tomato. Add cheese and beaten eggs. Season with salt and pepper. Cook on low heat. Lift occasionally from bottom of skillet with turner. When set but soft, stir in bacon.

Per serving (excluding unknown items): 206.8 Calories; 15.8 Fat (69.7 calories from fat); 14.4 Protein; 1.0 Carbohydrate; 298 Cholesterol; 320 Sodium.

Cream Cheese & Tomato Omelet

Makes 4 servings.

6 eggs
1/4 cup heavy cream
salt
black pepper
1/4 cup butter
6 ounces cream cheese cubed
2 whole fresh tomatoes peeled and chopped

Beat eggs until light, then beat in cream, salt, and pepper. Melt butter in a large skillet. Pour eggs into skillet. When set, but still soft, spread tomatoes and cheese over top. Fold in half. When bottom is brown, flip over and brown other side.

Per serving (excluding unknown items): 409.4 Calories; 38.3 Fat (83.0 calories from fat); 12.2 Protein; 5.5 Carbohydrate; 372 Cholesterol; 333 Sodium.

Pancakes

Makes 4 servings.

1 cup ricotta cheese
1/2 cup soy flour
1/4 cup wheat bran
1/2 teaspoon salt
1/8 teaspoon baking powder
1/4 cup heavy cream
4 large eggs
2 teaspoons oil
2 packets Sweet 'n Low® sweetener

Combine all dry ingredients in a mixing bowl and stir. Add ricotta, eggs and oil. With an electric mixer, mix on lowest speed for about 10 seconds and then at highest speed for about a minute. Coat griddle with vegetable spray and heat. Pour batter onto hot griddle to about a three-inch circle. Cook until bubbles surface on uncooked side, flip and cook until done. Serve with butter and sugar-free syrup.

Per serving (excluding unknown items): 298.1 Calories; 22.4 Fat (65.7 calories from fat); 16.8 Protein; 9.4 Carbohydrate; 235 Cholesterol; 392 Sodium.

Cheese Omelet In Microwave

Makes 2 servings.

3 large eggs
1/3 cup mayonnaise
2 tablespoons margarine
1/2 cup cheddar cheese shredded
chives
black olives chopped

Place the egg whites into a large mixing bowl. Beat at high speed until soft peaks form. In smaller bowl place the egg yolks, and using same beaters, beat yolks, mayonnaise and 2 tablespoons water. Gently pour yolk mixture over whites and fold in carefully. Melt margarine in 9-inch pie plate and swirl to coat inside. Carefully pour eggs into pie plate. Microwave at medium (half power) for 5 to 7 minutes. Sprinkle the shredded cheese over eggs and microwave at medium for 30 seconds to 1 minute. Sprinkle with chopped chives, olives, then quickly run a spatula around sides and bottom of dish. Fold half of omelet over the other half. Slide onto serving plate.

Per serving (excluding unknown items): 573.3 Calories; 58.3 Fat (88.7 calories from fat); 15.5 Protein; 1.3 Carbohydrate; 317 Cholesterol; 598 Sodium.

Eggs in Bacon Rings

Makes 3 servings.

6 slices bacon
6 eggs
salt and pepper

Curl slices of bacon around the inside of muffin pan. Break an egg into each cup within the bacon ring. Season with salt and pepper. Bake until set, not hard. Remove from pan carefully so bacon remains fastened to egg. Arrange on platter.

Per serving (excluding unknown items): 199.6 Calories; 14.8 Fat (68.1 calories from fat); 14.5 Protein; 1.1 Carbohydrate; 377 Cholesterol; 309 Sodium.

Mexican Eggs

Makes 4 servings.

2 tablespoons butter
8 eggs slightly beaten
2 green onions chopped
1/2 bell pepper chopped
1 cup Monterey jack cheese grated

Saute onions and bell pepper in butter. Add eggs and stir. Just before eggs are cooked, add cheese. Top with sour cream and/or hot sauce.

Per serving (excluding unknown items): 307.0 Calories; 22.8 Fat (66.3 calories from fat); 18.9 Protein; 7.1 Carbohydrate; 407 Cholesterol; 318 Sodium.

Scrambled Eggs with Cream Cheese

Makes 2 servings.

1/4 stick butter
6 eggs
1/8 cup heavy cream
1 1/2 ounces cream cheese cut in 1/2" cubes
salt and pepper to taste
1/2 tablespoon chives

Melt butter. Cook eggs with cream and cream cheese on very low heat until cheese melts. Add chives.

Per serving (excluding unknown items): 328.2 Calories; 27.1 Fat (74.9 calories from fat); 17.9 Protein; 2.6 Carbohydrate; 597 Cholesterol; 244 Sodium.

Baked Eggs

Makes 2 servings.

6 eggs
1/2 cup American cheese grated
1/4 cup heavy cream
1/4 cup water
2 tablespoons butter
1/2 teaspoon mustard
salt and pepper to taste

Mix all ingredients and pour into well greased 8-inch square pan. Bake at 325 degrees for 25-30 minutes.
Optional: Add fried bacon that's been crumbed and chopped onion.

Per serving (excluding unknown items): 500.3 Calories; 44.1 Fat (79.3 calories from fat); 23.0 Protein; 2.9 Carbohydrate; 648 Cholesterol; 488 Sodium.

Huevos y Queso

Makes 2 servings.

4 eggs
salt and pepper to taste
2 ounces American cheese (Velveeta)
splash heavy cream
1 teaspoon picante sauce

Scramble eggs. Salt and pepper to taste. While eggs are cooking, place cheese, cream and picante in a bowl. Microwave on high, stirring midway through, for one minute or until cheese is melted. Mix thoroughly. Pour over scrambled eggs and serve.

Per serving (excluding unknown items): 233.8 Calories; 17.4 Fat (67.9 calories from fat); 16.9 Protein; 1.6 Carbohydrate; 393 Cholesterol; 310 Sodium.

Cheese and Chili Puff

Makes 10 servings.

1 pound cheddar cheese grated
1 pound monterey jack cheese grated
4 ounces green chili peppers chopped
1 cup sour cream
3 eggs slightly beaten
1 teaspoon salt
1/8 teaspoon pepper

Combine both cheeses with chopped green chilies. Spread evenly in a buttered baking dish. Mix sour cream and eggs with salt and pepper. Pour over cheese mixture. Bake uncovered 45 to 50 minutes at 350 degrees. Serve immediately.

Per serving (excluding unknown items): 423.9 Calories; 34.9 Fat (74.1 calories from fat); 24.9 Protein; 2.6 Carbohydrate; 153 Cholesterol; 767 Sodium.

Soup & Salad

Fresh Tomato Bisque

Makes 8 servings.

1 large onion chopped
1 medium celery stalk chopped
1 teaspoon basil dried
1 clove garlic finely chopped
2 tablespoons butter
1 1/2 teaspoons chicken bouillon granules
1/2 packet Sweet 'n Low® sweetener
6 large tomatoes peeled and seeded
1 tablespoon lemon juice
freshly ground pepper

Cook and stir onion, celery, basil and garlic in butter in 3-quart saucepan about five minutes or until onion is tender. Stir in bouillon granules, sweetener and tomatoes. Heat to boiling; reduce heat. Cover and simmer about 10 minutes or until tomatoes are tender. Place half of the mixture in blender container. Cover and process until smooth. Return to saucepan. Heat through if necessary. Stir in lemon juice; sprinkle with pepper. Garnish with thin pats of butter if desired.
(About 1/2 cup servings.)

Per serving (excluding unknown items): 61.2 Calories; 3.0 Fat (41.0 calories from fat); 1.2 Protein; 8.6 Carbohydrate; 8 Cholesterol; 205 Sodium.

Cheesy Broccoli Soup

Makes 5 servings.

2 cups fresh broccoli pieces
1 medium onion quartered
14 ounces chicken broth
1 cup whipping cream
2 tablespoons flour
dash pepper
1/4 cup processed American cheese

Combine broccoli, onion, half of chicken broth and seasonings in 2 quart glass bowl. Cover with plastic wrap. Microwave on high 8 to 9 minutes or until broccoli is tender. Let stand 5 minutes. Pour mixture into blender. Cover and process at medium speed until smooth. Return mixture to bowl. Combine whipping cream and flour until smooth. Blend into hot vegetable mixture. Add pepper. Microwave on high, uncovered, 3 to 4 minutes or until mixture boils and thickens, stirring twice. Stir in cheese until blended. Mix in remaining chicken broth. Heat until warm.

Per serving (excluding unknown items): 230.6 Calories; 20.4 Fat (77.7 calories from fat); 4.4 Protein; 8.8 Carbohydrate; 71 Cholesterol; 606 Sodium.

Lobster Bisque

Makes 8 servings.

1 small onion finely chopped
3 tablespoons butter
3 tablespoons four
1 tablespoon parsley snipped fresh
1/2 teaspoon salt
1/8 teaspoon pepper
1 cup heavy cream
1 cup water
1 cup chicken broth
1 1/4 cups lobster meat fresh or frozen

Cook and stir onion in butter in 3-quart saucepan over low heat until onion is tender. Stir in flour, parsley, salt and pepper. Cook, stirring constantly, until mixture is bubbly. Remove from heat. Stir in cream, water and broth. Heat to boiling, stirring constantly. Boil and stir one minute. Stir in lobster. Heat to boiling. Reduce heat. Cook about three minutes, stirring frequently, until lobster is white.
(Makes 8 servings 1/2 cup each.)

Per serving (excluding unknown items): 185.5 Calories; 16.0 Fat (76.8 calories from fat); 7.8 Protein; 3.1 Carbohydrate; 86 Cholesterol; 492 Sodium.

Grilled Chicken Salad

Makes 4 servings.

tablespoon lemon juice freshly squeezed
3 tablespoons soy sauce
2 cloves garlic peeled and chopped
1/8 teaspoon black pepper
1 teaspoon basil dried
4 chicken breasts without skin
1/2 large red onion cut into 1/8" slices
vegetable oil
4 cups lettuce
4 tablespoons blue cheese crumbed
1 tomato cored and cut
4 tablespoons lemon juice freshly squeezed
4 tablespoons balsamic vinegar
2 cloves garlic peeled
2 teaspoons basil dried

Whisk together the lemon juice, soy sauce, garlic, black pepper and basil in a large bowl and set aside.

Pound the chicken to a thickness of 1/4 inch. Transfer the chicken to the marinade bowl and cover. Marinate in the refrigerator for at least 30 minutes.

Preheat the grill or broiler. Place the onion rounds in a single layer on a baking sheet and cover lightly with vegetable oil; turn them over and lightly coat the other side. Remove the chicken from the marinade and place alongside the onion rings. Grill or broil the onion rounds and chicken for 5 minutes per side. Let the chicken cool a bit, then slice thinly.

Spread an even amount of lettuce on 4 plates. Scatter the onion rounds and sliced chicken on top. Sprinkle 1 tablespoon blue cheese over each. Garnish with tomato wedges.

Combine all the dressing ingredients (beginning with lemon juice) in a blender and mix at low speed until the garlic is finely chopped. Spoon dressing onto the salads or serve it on the side.

Per serving (excluding unknown items): 304.6 Calories; 5.0 Fat (15.2 calories from fat); 55.0 Protein; 7.9 Carbohydrate; 135 Cholesterol; 1021 Sodium.

Chicken Salad Supreme

Makes 4 servings.

3/4 cup mayonnaise
3 tablespoons Dijon mustard
2 cups chicken cooked and cubed
2 tablespoons pickle relish
3/4 cup celery chopped
2 eggs, hard-boiled diced
1 tablespoon onion minced

Combine mayonnaise and mustard. Toss dressing lightly with remaining ingredients. Chill. If desired, serve on a bed of lettuce.

Per serving (excluding unknown items): 501.4 Calories; 44.1 Fat (76.5 calories from fat); 24.8 Protein; 5.8 Carbohydrate; 171 Cholesterol; 544 Sodium.

Bacon-Lettuce-Tomato Salad

Makes 8 servings.

6 cups lettuce torn
1 large tomato cut into wedges
1 pound bacon cooked and crumbled
2 green onions sliced
2 large avocados peeled and mashed
1/2 cup sour cream
1/4 cup whipping cream
1/4 cup mayonnaise-type salad dressing
1 tablespoon lemon juice
1/2 teaspoon salt

Combine the lettuce, tomato, bacon and green onion. Serve with Avocado Dressing.
AVOCADO DRESSING: Place avocados, sour cream, whipping cream, salad dressing, lemon juice and salt in bowl. Beat on low speed with mixer until smooth.

Per serving (excluding unknown items): 488.6 Calories; 42.0 Fat (76.5 calories from fat); 19.7 Protein; 9.4 Carbohydrate; 67 Cholesterol; 1109 Sodium.

Crab Louis

Makes 4 servings.

1 can cream of celery soup, condensed
1/2 cup chili sauce
1/4 cup mayonnaise
2 tablespoons onion finely chopped
dash of pepper
1/4 cup heavy cream whipped
4 cups crab meat cooked, flaked
1 hard-boiled egg cut in wedges
1 tomato cut in wedges

Blend soup, chili sauce, mayonnaise, onion and pepper; fold in whipped cream. Add crab; chill. Place crab on bed of lettuce. Garnish with egg and tomato.

Per serving (excluding unknown items): 353.0 Calories; 22.8 Fat (57.8 calories from fat); 30.6 Protein; 6.9 Carbohydrate; 197 Cholesterol; 1029 Sodium.

Celebration Salad

Makes 6 servings.

2 cups chicken, cooked and diced
2 cups ham, cooked and diced
2 cans celery diced
1/2 cup almonds
1/2 cup mayonnaise
1 hard-boiled egg
2 tablespoons pimiento slices
6 lettuce leaves

Combine chicken, ham, celery, almonds and mayonnaise. Serve on lettuce leaves. Cut egg lengthwise into eighths. Garnish salad with egg wedges.

Per serving (excluding unknown items): 175.7 Calories; 18.9 Fat (90.3 calories from fat); 2.4 Protein; 2.1 Carbohydrate; 36 Cholesterol; 125 Sodium.

Basic Chicken Salad

Makes 8 servings.

3 cups chicken cooked and chopped
1/2 green pepper chopped
4 stalks celery chopped
1/4 cup sweet pickles chopped
1 tablespoon lemon juice
1/2 teaspoon dry mustard
1/2 cup mayonnaise
2 tablespoons chives minced

In a food processor fitted with a steel blade, combine chicken, green pepper, celery and pickles. Process until finely chopped. Mixture should hold together firmly before dressing is added. Place chicken mixture in a large bowl. Add lemon juice, mustard, mayonnaise and chives. Mix well. Cover and refrigerate several hours. Serve on bed of lettuce.

Per serving (excluding unknown items): 224.9 Calories; 16.5 Fat (64.4 calories from fat); 16.1 Protein; 4.3 Carbohydrate; 53 Cholesterol; 210 Sodium.

Cobb Salad

Makes 6 servings.

6 cups lettuce shredded
3 cups chicken cooked and chopped
2 medium tomatoes seeded and chopped
3/4 cup blue cheese crumbled
6 slices bacon crumbed
3 eggs, hard-boiled chopped

Place shredded lettuce in 6 salad bowls. Evenly divide the chicken, tomatoes, blue cheese, bacon and eggs among the bowls. Serve with French Dressing.

Per serving (excluding unknown items): 287.9 Calories; 15.9 Fat (50.3 calories from fat); 29.5 Protein; 5.9 Carbohydrate; 172 Cholesterol; 395 Sodium.

Lettuce Wedges with Creamy Topping

Makes 6 servings.

1 medium iceberg lettuce
3 ounces cream cheese softened
1 small carrot grated
1/2 cup sour cream
2 tablespoons bell pepper finely chopped
2 tablespoons cheddar cheese shredded
1 teaspoon lemon juice
1/2 teaspoon salt
1/4 teaspoon onion salt
paprika

Cut lettuce into 6 wedges. Place one lettuce wedge on each of six salad plates. Make three to four vertical cuts almost to bottom of each wedge if desired. Mix remaining ingredients except paprika; spoon onto wedges. Sprinkle with paprika.

Per serving (excluding unknown items): 117.1 Calories; 9.9 Fat (74.4 calories from fat); 3.3 Protein; 4.4 Carbohydrate; 27 Cholesterol; 323 Sodium.

Sauces & Dressings

Hollandaise Sauce

Makes 8 servings.

1 cup butter at room temperature
2 tablespoons fresh lemon juice
3 tablespoons water
3 egg yolks
salt
white pepper

Cut butter into 1" pieces. In a small, heavy saucepan combine lemon juice and 2 tablespoons water and reduce over high heat to about one tablespoon. Remove from heat and add 1 tablespoon cold water. Beat egg yolks lightly and whisk into lemon water. Over low heat, whisk in the butter, one piece at a time, making sure that each piece of butter is melted before adding more. Continue to whisk the sauce until it is thick. Add salt and pepper to taste.

Per serving (excluding unknown items): 223.9 Calories; 24.6 Fat (97.0 calories from fat); 1.3 Protein; 0.5 Carbohydrate; 141 Cholesterol; 234 Sodium.

Vegetable Sauce

Makes 6 servings.

1 cup sour cream
1/4 cup mayonnaise
2 tablespoons lemon juice
1/2 teaspoon salt
1/4 teaspoon hot sauce (Tabasco)

Combine all ingredients in a saucepan and heat gently; do not allow to boil. Spoon over vegetables when serving. Ideal with cooked fresh asparagus, broccoli, cabbage, cauliflower or green beans.

Per serving (excluding unknown items): 149.4 Calories; 15.8 Fat (91.3 calories from fat); 1.3 Protein; 2.1 Carbohydrate; 20 Cholesterol; 251 Sodium.

Alfredo Sauce

Makes 4 servings.

6 tablespoons unsalted butter
2/3 cup heavy cream
1/2 teaspoon salt
ground white pepper
dash ground nutmeg
1 cup Parmesan cheese freshly grated

Place butter and cream in large skillet over medium-low heat. Cook and stir until butter melts and mixture bubbles; cook and stir 2 minutes more. Stir in salt, pepper and nutmeg. Remove from heat. Gradually stir in cheese until thoroughly blended and smooth. Return briefly to heat to completely blend cheese. (Do not let sauce bubble or cheese will become lumpy and tough.)

Per serving (excluding unknown items): 389.2 Calories; 38.9 Fat (88.7 calories from fat); 9.3 Protein; 1.9 Carbohydrate; 119 Cholesterol; 656 Sodium.

French Dressing

Makes 6 servings.

1/2 cup salad oil
1/3 cup red wine vinegar
1 tablespoon lemon juice
1 teaspoon Worcestershire sauce
1/2 teaspoon salt
1/4 packet Sweet 'n Low® sweetener
1/2 teaspoon dry mustard
1/2 teaspoon pepper
1 clove garlic minced

In a screw-top jar combine all ingredients. Cover and shake well. Shake before serving. Makes about one cup.

Per serving (excluding unknown items): 165.6 Calories; 18.2 Fat (96.2 calories from fat); 0.1 Protein; 1.5 Carbohydrate; 0 Cholesterol; 186 Sodium.

Mayonnaise-Salsa Dressing

Makes 8 servings.

1/3 cup prepared mayonnaise
4 cloves garlic crushed
1/3 cup prepared mild or hot chunky salsa
1 tablespoon sweet pickle relish

In a blender puree mayonnaise and garlic until garlic is incorporated. Stir in salsa and pickle relish.

Per serving (excluding unknown items): 73.1 Calories; 8.0 Fat (89.9 calories from fat); 0.3 Protein; 1.7 Carbohydrate; 3 Cholesterol; 140 Sodium.

Avocado Dressing

Makes 8 servings.

2 large avocados peeled and mashed
1/2 cup sour cream
1/4 cup half and half
1/4 cup mayonnaise-type salad dressing
1 tablespoon lemon juice
1/2 teaspoon salt

Place avocados, sour cream, half and half, salad dressing, lemon juice and salt in bowl. Beat on low speed with mixer until smooth. Cover and chill several hours.

Per serving (excluding unknown items): 129.6 Calories; 12.0 Fat (79.3 calories from fat); 1.5 Protein; 5.6 Carbohydrate; 11 Cholesterol; 200 Sodium.

Main Meals

Hamburger Steak with Mushroom Gravy

Makes 8 servings.

2 pounds ground beef
1 envelope onion soup mix
1 egg
1 can cream of mushroom soup, condensed
1/2 can water

Mix ground beef with 1/2 envelope of dry onion soup mix and 1 egg. Form into thick patties. Brown in skillet. Pour off grease. Combine one can of cream of mushroom soup, the remaining 1/2 envelope of dry onion soup mix and 1/2 soup can of water. Pour of meat. Cover and simmer until done.

Per serving (excluding unknown items): 413.4 Calories; 33.8 Fat (74.4 calories from fat); 20.7 Protein; 5.5 Carbohydrate; 120 Cholesterol; 830 Sodium.

Lasagna

Makes 8 servings.

1 1/2 pounds ground beef
1 jar spaghetti sauce
1 whole cabbage
12 ounces mozzarella cheese sliced

Brown ground beef and add spaghetti sauce. Separate the leaves of the cabbage. While sauce is simmering, steam cabbage leaves until tender. In a casserole dish layer cabbage leaves, sauce and mozzarella cheese slices, alternating until complete and ending with a last layer of cheese. Bake in 350 degree oven for 30 minutes or until cheese is melted.

Per serving (excluding unknown items): 449.0 Calories; 34.7 Fat (69.5 calories from fat); 25.1 Protein; 9.2 Carbohydrate; 110 Cholesterol; 407 Sodium.

Ranchero Supper Stew

Makes 6 servings.

2 tablespoons oil
1 1/2 pounds beef
1 envelope onion soup mix
16 ounces canned tomatoes undrained
1 cup water
2 teaspoons chili powder
1 carrot thinly sliced
1/2 green pepper chopped
1/4 cup celery thinly sliced

In large skillet, heat oil and brown beef; add onion soup mix blended with tomatoes, water and chili powder. Simmer for 30 minutes, stirring occasionally. Add carrots, green pepper and celery. Cook covered 45 minutes or until vegetables are tender and gravy is slightly thickened.

Per serving (excluding unknown items): 337.2 Calories; 24.7 Fat (65.8 calories from fat); 20.2 Protein; 8.8 Carbohydrate; 68 Cholesterol; 817 Sodium.

West Coast Broiled Flank Steak

Makes 4 servings.

1 1/2 pounds flank steak
1 onion thinly sliced
1 teaspoon lemon peel grated
1/2 cup lemon juice
3 packets Sweet 'n Low® sweetener
1/2 teaspoon salt
1/2 teaspoon oregano crushed
1/8 teaspoon coarse black pepper
1 tablespoon butter

Layer half of the onions in glass dish. Place steak on top of onions, cover with remaining onion. Thoroughly combine remaining ingredients except butter; pour over steak and onions. Marinate 2 to 3 hours or overnight in refrigerator, turning several times. Remove steak from marinade. Wipe partially dry with paper towel. Drain onions and reserve. Place steak on broiler pan 3 to 5 inches from source of heat. Broil 3 to 5 minutes on each side. Meanwhile, saute onions in butter until soft. To serve, cut steak across grain in very thin slices; top with onions.

Per serving (excluding unknown items): 396.1 Calories; 20.6 Fat (47.0 calories from fat); 45.7 Protein; 6.7 Carbohydrate; 94 Cholesterol; 418 Sodium.

Cabbage & Beef

Makes 6 servings.

1 1/2 pounds ground beef
1 large onion chopped
1 teaspoon seasoned salt
1/2 teaspoon salt
1/2 teaspoon pepper
1 can tomatoes with green chilis
1/2 cabbage chopped

Brown ground beef and onion in a large skillet. Season with salts and pepper. Add Rotel tomatoes. Stir in cabbage. Cover with a tight fitting lid and cook on low heat until cabbage is tender.

Per serving (excluding unknown items): 378.9 Calories; 30.4 Fat (72.3 calories from fat); 20.3 Protein; 5.9 Carbohydrate; 96 Cholesterol; 656 Sodium.

Herb-Marinated Chuck Steak

Makes 4 servings.

1 pound boneless beef chuck shoulder steak cut into 1" pieces
1/4 cup minced onion
2 tablespoons chopped fresh parsley
2 tablespoons white vinegar
1 tablespoon vegetable oil
2 teaspoons Dijon-style mustard
1 clove garlic crushed
1/2 teaspoon dried thyme leaves crushed

Combine onion, parsley, vinegar, oil, mustard, garlic and thyme. Place beef chuck shoulder steak in plastic bag; add marinade, turning to coat. Close bag securely and marinate in refrigerator 6 to 8 hours (or overnight, if desired), turning occasionally. Remove steak from marinade; discard marinade. Place steak on rack in broiler pan so surface of meat is 3 to 5 inches from heat. Broil steak 16 to 18 minutes for medium-rare to medium, turning once. Trim excess fat from steak.

Per serving (excluding unknown items): 273.4 Calories; 21.3 Fat (70.9 calories from fat); 18.2 Protein; 1.5 Carbohydrate; 66 Cholesterol; 127 Sodium.

Mexican Hamburgers

Makes 4 servings.

2 pounds ground beef
1 onion sliced
4 slices American cheese
1 jalapeno chopped
3 tablespoons oil (1 pound)
1 tablespoon flour
2 cups water

Form the ground beef into eight patties. Place on four of the patties one slice of onion, one slice of cheese and some chopped jalapeno. Place remaining four patties on top. Seal edges well. Place in skillet and brown on both sides. It will make its own oil or juice. Remove patties from skillet and make gravy as follows. Place in skillet three tablespoons of oil and one tablespoon of flour. Brown. Gradually add two cups of water. Stir until slightly thickened. Add patties. Cook 20 to 30 minutes longer. Turn patties over and cook 15 more minutes.

Per serving (excluding unknown items): 1244.2 Calories; 106.0 Fat (77.1 calories from fat); 63.6 Protein; 7.3 Carbohydrate; 300 Cholesterol; 897 Sodium.

Roast and Gravy

Makes 8 servings.

4 pounds roast
salt and pepper
1 can cream of mushroom soup, condensed
1 envelope onion soup mix

Tear foil enough to completely wrap chuck roast. Sprinkle roast with a little salt and pepper. Place roast on foil and spread with cream of mushroom soup and sprinkle with onion soup mix. wrap tightly and place in pan. Bake in preheated 300 degree oven for 2-1/2 to 3 hours. Roast makes gravy while cooking.

Per serving (excluding unknown items): 526.3 Calories; 38.6 Fat (67.2 calories from fat); 36.9 Protein; 5.4 Carbohydrate; 132 Cholesterol; 859 Sodium.

Crockpot Beef Stew

Makes 6 servings.

1 1/2 pounds beef roast
1/2 teaspoon black pepper
2 garlic cloves minced
1/2 package onion soup mix
2 teaspoons Worcestershire sauce
1 teaspoon steak sauce
3 carrots sliced
2 celery stalks diced
1 green bell pepper chopped
1 yellow onion
1/2 cup water
1/2 cup tomato juice

Cut roast into small portions and brown in a bit of oil. Slice onion and peppers and dice carrots and celery. Place in bottom of crockpot. Sprinkle beef pieces with fresh ground black pepper, minced garlic and the onion soup mix. Place on top of the vegetables. Mix the steak sauce and Worcestershire sauce with the water and tomato juice. Pour over meat. Cook on low for 7-9 hours. When ready to serve, dip meat and vegetables out of pot with a slotted spoon. Use the liquid as is or thicken with a little cornstarch.

Per serving (excluding unknown items): 277.1 Calories; 18.0 Fat (58.9 calories from fat); 19.2 Protein; 9.1 Carbohydrate; 66 Cholesterol; 473 Sodium.

Swiss Steak

Makes 4 servings.

1 1/2 pounds round steak
1 tablespoon vegetable shortening
1/2 cup canned tomatoes chopped
1/4 cup onion chopped
1/4 cup water
dash of pepper

Pound steak; cut into serving-size pieces. In heavy skillet, brown steak in shortening; pour off fat. Add remaining ingredients. Cover; simmer 1-1/2 hours or until done. Stir often.

Per serving (excluding unknown items): 362.6 Calories; 23.8 Fat (60.5 calories from fat); 33.0 Protein; 2.0 Carbohydrate; 101 Cholesterol; 140 Sodium.

Hamburger Gumbo

Makes 4 servings.

2 packages frozen okra
1/2 medium onion chopped
1 tablespoon butter
1 pound ground beef
4 ounces tomato sauce
4 ounces water
garlic powder
1 tablespoon chili powder
salt and pepper to taste

Saute onions in butter. Add meat and brown. Add okra and brown two minutes. Add all other ingredients and simmer 15 to 30 minutes, covered.

Per serving (excluding unknown items): 417.5 Calories; 33.5 Fat (71.8 calories from fat); 20.8 Protein; 8.9 Carbohydrate; 104 Cholesterol; 300 Sodium.

Texas Barbecue Beef Brisket

Makes 12 servings.

7 pounds boneless beef brisket
2 teaspoons paprika
1 teaspoon black pepper
1 medium onion grated
1 tablespoon butter
1 1/2 cups catsup
1 teaspoon fresh lemon juice
1 tablespoon Worcestershire sauce
1 teaspoon hot pepper sauce

Prepare briquets. Trim excess fat from beef brisket. Combine paprika and 1/2 teaspoon pepper; rub evenly over surface of brisket. Place brisket, fat side down, in 11 1/2 x 9-inch disposable aluminum pan. Add 1 cup water. Cover pan tightly with aluminum foil. Place in center of grid over very low coals. Cover cooker and cook 5 hours, turning brisket over every 11/2 hours. Add additional water to pan, if needed. Periodically add just enough additional briquets to keep coals at very low temperature.

Remove brisket form pan; reserve pan drippings. Place brisket on grid, fat side down, directly over very low coals. Replace grill cover and continue cooking 30 minutes. Reserve 1 cup drippings. Melt butter in medium saucepan over medium heat. Add onions; cook until tender-crisp. Add reserved pan drippings, remaining 1/2 teaspoon pepper, catsup, lemon juice, Worcestershire sauce and pepper sauce; simmer approximately 15 minutes, stirring occasionally. Trim excess fat from brisket; carve brisket across the grain into thin slices. Pour sauce over meat.

Per serving (excluding unknown items): 521.0 Calories; 26.3 Fat (46.4 calories from fat); 58.3 Protein; 9.9 Carbohydrate; 185 Cholesterol; 519 Sodium.

Spaghetti Squash Casserole

Makes 8 servings.

1 medium spaghetti squash
1/2 stick butter
1/2 pound mozzarella cheese shredded
1 pound ground beef
1 jar spaghetti sauce

Preheat oven to 375 degrees. Pierce squash in several places to vent steam. Place squash in large foil-lined baking dish; bake 20 minutes. Turn squash over; cook 25 minutes more or until easily depressed with finger. Cut in half immediately to prevent further cooking. Scoop seeds from squash. Create strands from squash by combing strands from each half of rind with two forks. Transfer strands to casserole dish. Mix in 1/2 stick of butter until melted. Layer mozzarella cheese over the squash. Brown beef and stir in spaghetti sauce. When heated through, pour over cheese. Bake in oven for 30 to 45 minutes.

Per serving (excluding unknown items): 309.4 Calories; 24.3 Fat (70.9 calories from fat); 16.2 Protein; 6.3 Carbohydrate; 76 Cholesterol; 319 Sodium.

Cabbage Goulash

Makes 5 servings.

1 head cabbage
1 pound ground beef
1 can cream of mushroom soup
1/2 cup whipping cream
1/2 onion chopped fine

Brown beef and onion in frying pan. Slice cabbage into 1/4 inch strips. Lay cabbage over beef. Cover with soup and cream to make a sauce. Simmer until tender.

Per serving (excluding unknown items): 420.3 Calories; 35.0 Fat (74.5 calories from fat); 18.1 Protein; 8.8 Carbohydrate; 110 Cholesterol; 306 Sodium.

Cheesy Meaty Broccoli

Makes 6 servings.

1 package broccoli, frozen
1 pound ground beef
1 small onion chopped
salt and pepper
1 can cream of mushroom soup, condensed
1/2 pound American cheese grated

Cook frozen broccoli according to directions. Brown separately the ground beef and chopped onion. Salt and pepper to taste. Spread broccoli in greased 6x9-inch baking dish. Top with meat mixture. Cover with cream of mushroom soup. Sprinkle American cheese on top. Bake at 350 degrees until hot through and through.

Per serving (excluding unknown items): 450.6 Calories; 35.9 Fat (71.6 calories from fat); 23.4 Protein; 8.7 Carbohydrate; 101 Cholesterol; 721 Sodium.

Pizza Burgers

Makes 4 servings.

2 pounds ground beef
1 teaspoon seasoned salt
1 tablespoon chopped parsley
1/8 teaspoon basil
1/8 teaspoon oregano
2 eggs beaten
1 package pork skins crushed
1/4 cup olive oil
6 slices mozzarella cheese
6 tablespoons pizza sauce
3 tablespoons parmesan cheese grated

Preheat oven to 400 degrees. Mix beef with salt, parsley, basil and oregano. Shape into six patties. Dip patties into eggs, then coat with crushed pork skins. Saute patties in olive oil until well browned on both sides. Arrange in a shallow baking dish. They must not touch. Top each patty with slice of cheese. Pour on one tablespoon of pizza sauce to each. Sprinkle with Parmesan cheese. Bake until patties are done (about 20 minutes.)

Per serving (excluding unknown items): 1434.2 Calories; 119.9 Fat (75.7 calories from fat); 79.4 Protein; 7.3 Carbohydrate; 440 Cholesterol; 1460 Sodium.

Mushroom-Stuffed Steak

Makes 4 servings.

3 pounds boneless beef top sirloin steak
1 tablespoon olive oil
1 cup fresh mushrooms finely chopped
1/4 cup minced green onion
1 tablespoon dry red wine
1/4 teaspoon salt
1/4 teaspoon dried thyme
1/4 teaspoon pepper

Heat oil in nonstick skillet over medium-high heat. Add mushrooms and onion; cook 4 to 5 minutes or until vegetables are tender. Add wine and cook until evaporated. Stir in salt, thyme and pepper. Remove from heat; cool thoroughly. Trim excess fat from sirloin steak. To cut pocket in steak, make horizontal cut through center of steak, parallel to surface of meat, approximately 1 inch from each side. Cut to, but not through, opposite side. Spoon cooled stuffing into pocket, spreading evenly. Secure opening with wooden picks. Place steak on rack in broiler pan so surface of meat is 4 to 5 inches from heat. Broil about 30 minutes, turning once. Place on warm serving platter. Carve steak into 1/2-inch thick slices.

Per serving (excluding unknown items): 741.3 Calories; 52.1 Fat (64.7 calories from fat); 62.4 Protein; 1.5 Carbohydrate; 217 Cholesterol; 309 Sodium.

Beef Zucchini Cheese-It

Makes 8 servings.

1 pound ground beef
1 teaspoon salt
1/4 teaspoon pepper
1 clove garlic mashed
3 pounds zucchini
4 ounces chili peppers
2 tablespoons butter
1 cup cheddar cheese shredded
2 eggs
2 cups cottage cheese
2 tablespoons parmesan cheese grated

Cook meat in skillet. Spoon into casserole dish. Cook zucchini in salted water until tender. Drain well and mash. Whip in chiles, onion and butter. Spread over meat mixture and sprinkle with cheddar cheese. Beat eggs. Fold in cottage cheese. Spoon over zucchini. Sprinkle with Parmesan cheese. Bake 34 to 45 minutes until set.

Per serving (excluding unknown items): 357.7 Calories; 25.4 Fat (63.4 calories from fat); 24.7 Protein; 8.2 Carbohydrate; 122 Cholesterol; 694 Sodium.

Cheese-Filled Burgers

Makes 6 servings.

2 pounds ground beef
1 tablespoon chives chopped
2 teaspoons seasoned salt
1 small tomato diced
1 egg beaten
6 ounces cheddar cheese coarsely grated

Combine beef with all ingredients except cheese. Shape into 12 equal balls. Flatten each ball to pancake shape. Divide cheese into six piles and press together. Place 1 pile of cheese in center of six of the patties. Place second meat patty on top. Press edges together to seal. Grill, broil or saute with butter in a nonstick skillet.

Per serving (excluding unknown items): 595.3 Calories; 50.3 Fat (77.0 calories from fat); 33.1 Protein; 0.7 Carbohydrate; 188 Cholesterol; 743 Sodium.

Italian Sirloin Stew

Makes 4 servings.

1 pound sirloin steak cut 1 inch thick
1 large garlic clove crushed
2 tablespoons olive oil divided
1 medium onion cut 1/4 inch thick
1 teaspoon dried basil
1/8 teaspoon red pepper ground
1 14.5 oz can tomatoes undrained
1 cup beef broth
2 medium zucchini cut 1/4 inch slices

Cut beef steak into 1/4-inch thick strips; cut each strip into 1-inch pieces. Combine garlic with 1 tablespoon oil; stir into beef and reserve. Saute onion in remaining oil in large saucepan three minutes. Sprinkle with basil and pepper; cook and stir one minute. Add tomatoes, beef broth and zucchini. Bring to a boil; cover, reduce heat and simmer 15 minutes. Meanwhile, heat large nonstick skillet over medium-high heat. Cook and stir beef one to two minutes; add to sauce. Stir two teaspoons cornstarch dissolved in two tablespoons water into stew and cook until slightly thickened, about two minutes. Sprinkle with grated parmesan cheese.

Per serving (excluding unknown items): 336.2 Calories; 23.8 Fat (63.9 calories from fat); 22.4 Protein; 7.8 Carbohydrate; 73 Cholesterol; 455 Sodium.

Microwave Chili

Makes 6 servings.

1 pound ground beef
1 medium onion chopped
1 cup celery chopped
2 cans tomato soup
1/4 cup water
2 teaspoons chili powder
1 teaspoon brown sugar substitute
1 teaspoon Worcestershire sauce
1/2 teaspoon salt
1/2 teaspoon pepper
1/8 teaspoon cayenne pepper

Combine meat, onion and celery in three quart casserole dish. Microwave on high 6 to 9 minutes or until meat is cooked and vegetables are tender. Drain fat and break up meat. Stir in remaining ingredients. Cover. Microwave on high 5 minutes. Stir. Reduce power to 50 percent. Microwave uncovered 30 to 35 minutes, stirring twice. Makes two quarts.

Per serving (excluding unknown items): 279.1 Calories; 21.0 Fat (67.3 calories from fat); 13.8 Protein; 9.1 Carbohydrate; 64 Cholesterol; 553 Sodium.

Meatloaf

Makes 6 servings.

1 1/2 pounds ground beef
16 ounces tomato sauce
2 eggs
1/4 cup onion chopped
1/4 cup bell pepper chopped
1 cup cheddar cheese grated
1/4 teaspoon salt
1/4 teaspoon pepper
1/4 teaspoon garlic

Mix all ingredients well. Place in a loaf pan. Bake in 350 degree oven for 45 minutes.

Per serving (excluding unknown items): 476.9 Calories; 38.0 Fat (71.8 calories from fat); 26.5 Protein; 7.1 Carbohydrate; 177 Cholesterol; 759 Sodium.

Italian Goolaush

Makes 4 servings.

1 pound ground beef
1/2 zucchini julienned
1 can tomatoes diced
8 ounces ricotta cheese
1 small onion
garlic
oregano
salt and pepper
8 ounces mozzarella cheese shredded

Brown beef in a saucepan. Add tomatoes, onion, garlic and spices. Cook until onions are translucent. Add zucchini and entire container of ricotta cheese. Mix ingredients together and pour into a baking dish. Bake at 350 degrees for 20 to 30 minutes. Sprinkle mozzarella cheese on top and return to oven long enough to melt the cheese.

Per serving (excluding unknown items): 656.1 Calories; 51.6 Fat (71.1 calories from fat); 38.4 Protein; 8.9 Carbohydrate; 176 Cholesterol; 365 Sodium.

Ham and Cheese Chicken Rolls

Makes 6 servings.

4 boned and skinned chicken breast halves
4 slices cooked ham
4 slices Swiss cheese
2 tablespoons vegetable oil
10 ounces cream of chicken soup
1/3 cup whipping cream
1/4 cup green onions sliced

Flatten chicken to even thickness using palm of hand or flat side of meat mallet. Place one ham slice and one cheese slice on each breast half. Roll up chicken from narrow end, jelly-roll fashion. Tuck in ham and cheese, if necessary; secure with wooden toothpicks. In 10-inch skillet over medium-high heat, in hot oil, cook chicken rolls 10 minutes or until browned on all sides. Spoon off fat. Stir in soup, cream and onions. Heat to boiling. Reduce heat to low. Cover and cook 10 minutes or until chicken is no longer pink, stirring occasionally. Remove toothpicks and spoon some sauce over chicken rolls.

Per serving (excluding unknown items): 628.2 Calories; 42.2 Fat (61.1 calories from fat); 52.4 Protein; 7.9 Carbohydrate; 177 Cholesterol; 1660 Sodium.

Chicken with Cilantro Pesto

Makes 4 servings.

4 chicken breast, no skin, no bone
1/4 cup cilantro pesto (see recipe)
2 teaspoons cooking oil
1/4 teaspoon paprika

Place each chicken breast half between 2 pieces of clear plastic wrap. Pound lightly to 1/4-inch thickness. Remove plastic wrap. Spread one tablespoon Cilantro Pesto on each breast half. Roll up chicken, jelly-roll style. Secure with wooden toothpicks. Place chicken rolls in a shallow baking dish. Brush lightly with oil; sprinkle with paprika. Bake in a 375 degree oven for 25 to 30 minutes. If desired, serve with sour cream and additional Cilantro Pesto.

Per serving (excluding unknown items): 82.5 Calories; 7.7 Fat (80.8 calories from fat); 2.4 Protein; 1.7 Carbohydrate; 6 Cholesterol; 124 Sodium.

Cilantro Pesto

Makes 16 servings.

1 1/2 cups cilantro leaves
1/2 cup parsley sprigs stems removed
1/2 cup Asiago cheese grated
2 cloves garlic quartered
1/4 teaspoon salt
1/4 cup olive oil

In a blender or food processor combine cilantro, parsley, Asiago cheese (or Parmesan), garlic and salt. Cover and blend with several on-off turns till a paste forms, stopping the machine several times and scraping the sides. With machine running, gradually add the oil and blend or process to the consistency of soft butter. Serving size is one tablespoon.

Per serving (excluding unknown items): 65.1 Calories; 5.6 Fat (75.0 calories from fat); 2.5 Protein; 1.7 Carbohydrate; 7 Cholesterol; 130 Sodium.

Chicken Florentine

Makes 6 servings.

1/2 pound fresh spinach stems removed, wash
4 tablespoons butter
1 whole large onion cut into rings
2 whole chicken breasts cut into 2" pieces
6 ounces mushrooms sliced
1/3 cup dry white wine
1 tablespoon flour
1 cup sour cream
1 pinch garlic powder
4 ounces sharp cheddar cheese grated

Steam spinach until wilted, drain and chop. Melt 2 tablespoons of butter in large skillet and saute onions until golden. Remove onions with slotted spoon, mix with spinach and place in buttered casserole. Add 1 tablespoon butter to skillet. Brown chicken and remove to warm plate. Saute mushrooms in remaining butter and remove to plate with chicken. Add wine to pan and then stir in flour. Slowly add sour cream and stir until hot and thickened. Add chicken, mushrooms, and garlic powder. Place on spinach, sprinkle with cheese and bake uncovered at 350 for 20 to 30 minutes.

Per serving (excluding unknown items): 427.9 Calories; 31.0 Fat (61.7 calories from fat); 35.8 Protein; 7.5 Carbohydrate; 139 Cholesterol; 300 Sodium.

Basil Grilled Chicken

Makes 4 servings.

3/4 teaspoon pepper coarsely ground
4 chicken breasts without skin
1/3 cup butter melted
1/4 cup fresh basil chopped
1/2 cup butter softened
2 tablespoons fresh basil minced
1 tablespoon Parmesan cheese grated
1/4 teaspoon garlic powder
1/8 teaspoon salt
1/8 teaspoon pepper

Press 3/4 teaspoon pepper into meaty sides of chicken breast halves. Combine 1/3 cup melted butter and 1/4 cup chopped basil; stir well. Brush chicken lightly with melted butter mixture.

Combine 1/2 cup softened butter, 2 tablespoons basil, Parmesan cheese, garlic powder, salt and pepper in small bowl. Beat at low speed of an electric mixer until mixture is well blended and smooth. Transfer to a small serving bowl; set aside.

Grill chicken over medium coals 8 to 10 minutes on each side, basting frequently with remaining melted butter mixture. Serve grilled chicken with basil-butter mixture.

Per serving (excluding unknown items): 589.0 Calories; 41.0 Fat (63.4 calories from fat); 52.8 Protein; 0.6 Carbohydrate; 233 Cholesterol; 622 Sodium.

Chicken Ole'

Makes 6 servings.

1/2 cup picante sauce medium hot
1/4 cup dijon mustard
2 tablespoons lime juice
3 whole chicken breasts skinned and boned
2 tablespoons butter

Combine picante sauce, mustard and lime juice in large bowl. Add chicken, turning to coat. Cover; marinate in refrigerator at least 30 minutes. Melt butter in large skillet over medium heat until foamy. Remove chicken from marinade; reserve marinade. Add chicken to skillet; cook about 10 minutes or until brown on both sides. Add marinade; cook about 5 minutes or until chicken is tender and marinade glazes chicken. Remove chicken to serving platter. Boil marinade over high heat 1 minute. Pour over chicken.

Per serving (excluding unknown items): 297.4 Calories; 18.0 Fat (47.3 calories from fat); 42.7 Protein; 2.4 Carbohydrate; 133 Cholesterol; 400 Sodium.

Marinated Italian Garlic Chicken

Makes 4 servings.

4 chicken breast halves
1/2 cup mayonnaise-type salad dressing
1/2 cup Italian salad dressing
1/4 teaspoon garlic powder
1/8 teaspoon ground red pepper

Mix dressings and seasonings. Pour dressing mixture over chicken. Cover; refrigerate 20 minutes. Drain. Place chicken on grill over medium-hot coals or greased rack of broiler pan. Grill or broil for 10 to 12 minutes on each side or until tender.

Per serving (excluding unknown items): 501.6 Calories; 37.4 Fat (61.5 calories from fat); 42.5 Protein; 10.2 Carbohydrate; 131 Cholesterol; 531 Sodium.

Cozy Lime Chicken For Two

Makes 2 servings.

4 favorite broiler-fryer chicken parts
4 tablespoons fresh lime juice
2 tablespoons olive oil
1/2 teaspoon salt
1/2 teaspoon freshly ground pepper
3 ounces sliced mushrooms in butter

In small bowl, mix lime juice and olive oil. Dip each chicken part in mixture, covering completely. On foil-lined baking pan, arrange chicken in single layer; sprinkle with salt and pepper. Arrange oven rack at least 6 inches from heat and set temperature at broil (450F.). Broil chicken about 15 minutes; turn and pour remaining lime-oil mixture over chicken. Continue to broil about 15 minutes more or until fork can be inserted in chicken with ease. Pour mushrooms in butter from can over chicken and return to oven for about 2 minutes or until mushrooms are hot.

Per serving (excluding unknown items): 453.3 Calories; 35.5 Fat (70.8 calories from fat); 28.0 Protein; 5.0 Carbohydrate; 133 Cholesterol; 638 Sodium.

Chicken Souffleé

Makes 4 servings.

1 can cream of mushroom soup, condensed
1/2 cup light cream
4 eggs separated
1 egg white
1 cup chicken shredded

Heat soup in a double boiler top while separating the eggs. Beat the egg yolks until thick and lemon-colored.

Remove the soup pot and add egg yolks, stirring well. Add chicken. Cool slightly. Beat 5 egg whites until very stiff. Fold into egg yolk mixture. Gently turn the batter into a well-buttered souffle dish and bake at 375 degrees for 30 minutes.

Per serving (excluding unknown items): 279.8 Calories; 18.9 Fat (61.6 calories from fat); 18.7 Protein; 7.9 Carbohydrate; 236 Cholesterol; 728 Sodium.

Tempting Tomato Chicken Grill

Makes 4 servings.

4 broiler-fryer chicken quarters
1/4 cup fresh lime juice
1 1/2 teaspoons chopped chives
1 teaspoon freshly grated ginger
2 cloves garlic minced
2 tablespoons olive oil
1 teaspoon chili powder
1 cup medium salsa chunky style

In small saucepan, mix together lime juice, chives, ginger and garlic. Add olive oil and chili powder and heat to boiling over medium heat (or in microwave if glass dish is used). Stir in salsa. Place chicken in single layer in large, shallow bowl. Pour sauce over chicken and turn to coat well. Cover and refrigerate at least 2 hours. When ready to cook, place chicken on prepared grill, skin side up, about 8 inches from heat. Grill, turning every 10 minutes, about 1 hour or until fork can be inserted in chicken with ease. Heat marinade to boiling and boil about 3 minutes; pour over chicken.

Per serving (excluding unknown items): 243.0 Calories; 18.7 Fat (67.4 calories from fat); 14.3 Protein; 6.1 Carbohydrate; 66 Cholesterol; 494 Sodium.

Chicken Fajitas

Makes 4 servings.

6 boned and skinned chicken breast halves sliced
1 red pepper
1 onion
1 green pepper
oil
--MARINADE--
1 clove garlic
1 1/2 teaspoons seasoned salt
1/2 teaspoon crushed red pepper
1/2 teaspoon chili powder
2 tablespoons oil
2 tablespoons fresh lemon juice
1 1/2 teaspoons cumin

Mix marinade and pour in zip-lock bag. Place chicken in bag. Let marinate for a minimum of four hours. Stir fry onion in oil until soft and then add chicken and rest of vegetables and stir fry until done.

Per serving (excluding unknown items): 236.8 Calories; 8.8 Fat (34.1 calories from fat); 31.5 Protein; 7.0 Carbohydrate; 77 Cholesterol; 605 Sodium.

Baked Buffalo Wings

Makes 4 servings.

2 tablespoons melted butter
1/4 cup hot pepper sauce
2 tablespoons rice vinegar
30 chicken drumettes
paprika for sprinkling
-----Roquefort Dressing-----
6 ounces Roquefort cheese
1 cup sour cream
2 tablespoons mayonnaise
freshly ground pepper to taste

Preheat oven to 350 degrees. Lightly oil a baking sheet. Mix together butter, hot-pepper sauce and vinegar. Dip chicken into mixture, then place on prepared baking sheet. Sprinkle lightly with paprika. Bake until crisp and brown (about 30 minutes). Serve with celery sticks and Roquefort Dressing.

ROQUEFORT DRESSING: Mix Roquefort, sour cream, and mayonnaise together. Season with pepper.

Per serving (excluding unknown items): 1192.8 Calories; 94.9 Fat (72.1 calories from fat); 78.1 Protein; 4.7 Carbohydrate; 362 Cholesterol; 1166 Sodium.

Pizza Chicken Italiano

Makes 4 servings.

4 boned and skinned chicken breasts
8 ounces tomato sauce
1 1/2 teaspoons oregano
1 teaspoon chopped parsley
1/2 teaspoon garlic salt
1/2 teaspoon onion powder
1/4 package Sweet 'n Low® sweetener
4 slices mozzarella cheese

Place chicken in 2-quart baking dish. Combine tomato sauce, oregano, chopped parsley, garlic salt, onion powder and sweetener. Pour over chicken, cover and bake at 425 degrees for 15 minutes. Top with Mozzarella cheese and continue to bake, uncovered, for 10 minutes.

Per serving (excluding unknown items): 564.3 Calories; 30.1 Fat (48.7 calories from fat); 63.7 Protein; 7.7 Carbohydrate; 198 Cholesterol; 1178 Sodium.

Double-Delicious Chicken Souffle

Makes 6 servings.

4 eggs
1 can cream of chicken soup
1 teaspoon curry powder
2/3 teaspoon salt
1/2 pepper
2 cups chicken cooked and diced
2 tablespoons butter
2 tablespoons flour
1/2 cup heavy cream
1/2 cup water
1/4 cup Swiss cheese grated
1/8 teaspoon cream of tartar

Preheat oven to 375 degrees. Place oven rack at center position. Lightly butter a 1-1/2 quart round baking dish. Refrigerate dish until butter is firm. Separate eggs, placing yolks in small bowl and whites in a large bowl; set aside. In a medium bowl, combine chicken soup, curry powder and 1/4 teaspoon salt. Season with pepper. Add chicken; stir until blended. Spoon into buttered dish; set aside. Melt two tablespoons of butter over low heat in a large saucepan. Stir in flour; cook until frothy. Slowly add cream/water, stirring constantly until it becomes a smooth thick sauce. Remove from heat. Season with 1/2 teaspoon salt and 1/4 teaspoon pepper. Beat in egg yolks.

Stir in cheese; set aside until slightly cooled, stirring occasionally to keep a film from forming over surface. Beat egg whites until frothy. Add cream of tartar; beat until soft peaks from. Using a spatula, fold about 1/4 of beaten egg whites into cheese mixture. Gently fold cheese mixture into remaining beaten egg whites. Spoon over chicken in baking dish. Bake 30 to 35 minutes or until lightly browned and set in the center.

Per serving (excluding unknown items): 293.6 Calories; 20.8 Fat (64.1 calories from fat); 20.2 Protein; 6.0 Carbohydrate; 208 Cholesterol; 538 Sodium.

Lime & Honey Broiled Chicken

Makes 2 servings.

2 broiler-fryer chicken quarters
1/4 cup fresh lime juice
1 tablespoon butter
1 teaspoon honey
1/4 teaspoon garlic powder
2 tablespoons white wine
1/2 teaspoon salt
1/4 teaspoon coarsely ground pepper

In small saucepan, place lime juice, butter, honey and garlic powder. Heat over high temperature until margarine melts, about 2 minutes. Add white wine and stir to mix. Line a small baking pan (just large enough to hold chicken) with foil; arrange chicken in pan, skin side up. Pour lime juice sauce over chicken and let stand 5 minutes. Sprinkle with salt and pepper. Set oven temperature control at broil (450 F.) and arrange rack so chicken is about 5 inches from heat. Broil 15 minutes; turn chicken and spoon sauce from pan over chicken. Broil about 15 minutes more or until fork can be inserted in chicken with ease. Remove from oven; spoon sauce from pan over chicken and let stand about 3 minutes.

Per serving (excluding unknown items): 238.1 Calories; 16.6 Fat (65.1 calories from fat); 13.8 Protein; 6.2 Carbohydrate; 82 Cholesterol; 644 Sodium.

Crispy Buttered Wings

Makes 2 servings.

24 chicken wings
1 stick butter
salt and pepper
garlic

Fold wing tips in. Place wings in casserole dish. Cut butter into squares and place all over wings. Season heavily with salt, pepper and garlic. Place in oven preheated to 400 degrees. Cook for 30 minutes. Remove and flip wings over. Cook additional 20 minutes or until crisp.

Per serving (excluding unknown items): 1344.8 Calories; 98.8 Fat (67.5 calories from fat); 107.0 Protein; 0.0 Carbohydrate; 464 Cholesterol; 484 Sodium.

Grilled Chicken & Green Bean Salad

Makes 8 servings.

5 boneless skinless chicken breasts
1 red bell pepper cut in 1/4" strips
1 green bell pepper cut in 1/4" strips
1 small red onion cut in 1/4" strips
strips
1/2 pound fresh green beans snapped and blanched
--DRESSING--
1 cup mayonnaise
6 ounces mustard creole style
1 teaspoon cider vinegar
1 package Sweet 'n Low® sweetener
1/2 teaspoon salt
1/4 teaspoon white pepper

Place chicken on prepared grill and cook about 5 minutes per side. Chill in refrigerator; cut into 1/4-inch strips. In large mixing bowl, place chicken, peppers, onion and green beans. To prepare dressing, in medium bowl, mix together 1 cup mayonnaise, 1 jar (6 oz.) Creole mustard, 1 teaspoon cider vinegar, 1 package sweetener, 1/2 teaspoon salt and 1/4 teaspoon white pepper. Add dressing and toss gently to mix well.

Per serving (excluding unknown items): 351.3 Calories; 26.1 Fat (64.6 calories from fat); 26.2 Protein; 6.0 Carbohydrate; 70 Cholesterol; 629 Sodium.

Baked Cornish Game Hens

Makes 6 servings.

6 whole Cornish game hens
1 medium onion chopped
1 celery stalk chopped
1/2 green pepper chopped
8 ounces mushrooms chopped
1 whole garlic clove minced
2 tablespoons fresh basil minced
1 teaspoon oregano
2 tablespoons fresh parsley
3/4 cup butter melted

Stir 1/2 cup melted butter with onion, celery, green pepper, mushrooms, garlic and herbs. Season hens inside and out with salt and pepper. Stuff bird with equal amounts of the vegetable mix. Place birds in baking dish, breast side up. Drizzle with remaining 1/4 cup butter. Cover and bake 1-1/2 hours at 325 degrees. Brown at 500 degrees.

Per serving (excluding unknown items): 1570.7 Calories; 99.6 Fat (58.3 calories from fat); 155.4 Protein; 4.8 Carbohydrate; 356 Cholesterol; 608 Sodium.

Frittata di Pollo

Makes 4 servings.

6 eggs
1/2 teaspoon salt
1/4 teaspoon pepper coarsely ground
1/2 cup chicken cooked and diced
2 slices salami cut in narrow strips
1/4 cup zucchini thinly sliced
1/4 cup Parmesan cheese grated
1 tablespoon butter
2 tablespoons vegetable oil

Place oven rack 2 inches below heat. Preheat broiler to high. In a large bowl, beat eggs until blended. Add salt, pepper, chicken, salami, zucchini and cheese. Heat butter and oil in a 12-inch ovenproof skillet over medium heat until foamy. When foam subsides, add egg mixture. Reduce heat to low. Cook egg mixture 10 minutes, sliding skillet back and forth over heat until eggs have set on the bottom but are still moist on top. Place skillet under broiler, leaving oven door open. Broil until top is puffy and firm. Using a spatula, loosen frittata and slide onto a platter. Cut into wedges. Serve warm, topped with pizza sauce, if desired.

Per serving (excluding unknown items): 277.5 Calories; 22.0 Fat (71.9 calories from fat); 17.4 Protein; 1.9 Carbohydrate; 312 Cholesterol; 636 Sodium.

Chicken Alfredo

Makes 4 servings.

4 boned and skinned chicken breast halves
3 tablespoons butter
1/4 teaspoon salt and pepper each
1/8 teaspoon garlic
1 serving Alfredo Sauce (see recipe)
8 slices bacon fried and crumbled

Prepare Alfredo Sauce. In a skillet melt three tablespoons of butter. Season chicken breasts with salt, pepper and garlic. Place chicken in skillet and fry in butter until done. Place chicken breast on plate, sprinkle with bacon crumbles and pour 1/4 of Alfredo sauce on top. Serve.

Per serving (excluding unknown items): 342.6 Calories; 25.6 Fat (66.7 calories from fat); 26.6 Protein; 2.2 Carbohydrate; 115 Cholesterol; 599 Sodium.

Chicken Divan

Makes 4 servings.

2 chicken breasts split
1 package frozen broccoli spears
4 ounces processed American cheese
1 can cream of mushroom soup
1/2 teaspoon salt
1/4 teaspoon rosemary
1/8 teaspoon pepper
1 teaspoon Worcestershire sauce
2 tablespoons chicken broth

Place chicken breasts in microwave-safe baking dish. Cover with waxed paper. Microwave on medium 12 to 14 minutes or until tender. Uncover and allow to cool. Microwave on high broccoli 8 to 9 minutes or until thawed. Drain and set aside. Remove chicken from baking dish. Remove skin and bones. Cut chicken into pieces. Arrange broccoli in baking dish and top with chicken. Crumble cheese over chicken. Combine soup, salt, rosemary, pepper, Worcestershire sauce and broth; pour over chicken. Microwave on high, uncovered, 8 minutes. Then microwave on medium 4 to 6 minutes until heated in center.

Per serving (excluding unknown items): 411.0 Calories; 24.8 Fat (49.0 calories from fat); 51.1 Protein; 6.9 Carbohydrate; 151 Cholesterol; 1094 Sodium.

Picante Chicken

Makes 3 servings.

1 medium lime
1/2 cup picante sauce
3 whole skinless boneless chicken breasts
2 tablespoons butter

Juice the lime. Combine lime juice, picante sauce and mustard in large bowl. Add chicken, turning to coat with marinade. Cover; marinate in refrigerator at least 30 minutes. Melt butter in large skillet until foamy. Drain chicken, reserving marinade. Add chicken to skillet in single layer. Cook 10 minutes or until chicken is lightly browned on both sides. Add reserved marinade to skillet; cook 5 minutes or until chicken is tender and glazed with marinade. Remove chicken to serving platter. Boil marinade in skillet over high heat 1 minute; pour over chicken.

Per serving (excluding unknown items): 267.1 Calories; 10.3 Fat (34.9 calories from fat); 38.8 Protein; 4.5 Carbohydrate; 117 Cholesterol; 476 Sodium.

Glorified Chicken Bake

Makes 4 servings.

1 whole frying chicken cut up
1 tablespoon butter melted
10 ounces cream of chicken soup

In oblong baking dish, arrange chicken skin-side up. Drizzle with melted butter. Bake at 375 degrees for 40 minutes. Spoon soup over chicken. Bake 20 minutes more or until chicken is no longer pink and juice runs clear.

Per serving (excluding unknown items): 490.3 Calories; 22.9 Fat (43.4 calories from fat); 61.2 Protein; 6.0 Carbohydrate; 196 Cholesterol; 494 Sodium.

Baked Fresh Ham

Makes 12 servings.

10 pounds fresh ham
2 whole garlic clove minced
2 tablespoons olive oil
1/2 teaspoon dried rosemary
1/2 teaspoon ground thyme
1 cup light beer

Trim excess fat from ham. Mix oil with herbs and rub all over ham. Bake at 350 degrees for 30-35 minutes per pound of meat, until meat thermometer registers 185 degrees. Baste occasionally with beer.

Per serving (excluding unknown items): 723.5 Calories; 51.5 Fat (66.1 calories from fat); 58.9 Protein; 0.5 Carbohydrate; 207 Cholesterol; 192 Sodium.

Barbecued Pork Southern Style

Makes 6 servings.

3 pounds pork shoulder roast
1 teaspoon celery seed
1/3 cup cider vinegar
1/2 cup ketchup
1/2 teaspoon chili powder
1/2 teaspoon ground nutmeg
1 teaspoon brown sugar
1/8 teaspoon ground cinnamon
1 bay leaf crumbled
1/2 teaspoon salt
1/2 teaspoon lemon pepper
1 dash hot pepper sauce
1 cup water

Brown the roast on all sides in a small amount of oil. Place the roast in an oven-safe pan with tight fitting lid or seal with aluminum foil. Place the remaining ingredients in a saucepan and bring to a boil. Boil for 1 minute; pour mixture over the roast. Cover tightly. Place the roast in a preheated 325-degree oven and bake for about 35-45 minutes per pound. Baste several times with the juices in the pan.

Per serving (excluding unknown items): 431.9 Calories; 30.9 Fat (65.0 calories from fat); 29.7 Protein; 7.7 Carbohydrate; 121 Cholesterol; 558 Sodium.

Chili-Marinated Pork

Makes 4 servings.

3 tablespoons ground seeded dried pasilla chilies
1 teaspoon coarse salt
1/2 teaspoon ground cumin
2 tablespoons vegetable oil
1 tablespoon fresh lime juice
3 cloves garlic minced
2 pounds pork tenderloin

Mix chilies, salt and cumin in small bowl. Stir in oil and lime juice to make smooth paste. Stir in garlic. Cut tenderloin crosswise into 8 equal pieces. Place pork between pieces of plastic wrap. Pound with flat side of mallet into 1/4-inch thickness. Spread chili paste on both sides of pork pieces to coat evenly. Place in shallow glass baking dish. Marinate for 2 to 3 hours. Prepare coals for grill. Grill pork 8 to 10 minutes, turning once.

Per serving (excluding unknown items): 338.8 Calories; 14.7 Fat (40.2 calories from fat); 47.9 Protein; 1.2 Carbohydrate; 148 Cholesterol; 585 Sodium.

Quiche Lorraine

Makes 4 servings.

12 slices bacon fried and crumbled
1 cup Swiss cheese shredded
1/3 cup onion minced
4 eggs
2 cups whipping cream
3/4 teaspoon salt
1/4 teaspoon sugar substitute
1/8 teaspoon cayenne pepper

Heat oven to 425 degrees. You must use a very good non-stick pie pan. Sprinkle bacon, cheese and onion in pie pan. Beat eggs slightly. Beat in remaining ingredients. Pour mixture into pie pan. Bake 15 minutes. Reduce oven temperature to 300 degrees. Bake 30 minutes longer.

Per serving (excluding unknown items): 695.3 Calories; 65.4 Fat (84.0 calories from fat); 21.8 Protein; 6.2 Carbohydrate; 388 Cholesterol; 876 Sodium.

Creamy Blue Cheese & Chicken Quiche

Makes 8 servings.

8 ounces cream cheese
1/2 cup heavy cream
1/2 cup water
1/2 cup blue cheese crumbled
4 eggs
1 cup chicken cooked and cubed
1/4 cup bacon crumbled
2 ounces pimientos drained
salt and pepper to taste

Preheat oven to 375 degrees. In a saucepan, combine cream cheese and cream/water. Stir over low heat until smooth. Stir in blue cheese. Gradually add cheese mixture to eggs, stirring with a whisk as added. Add chicken, bacon and pimientos. Season to taste with salt and pepper. Pour into a non-stick pie pan. Bake 40 to 45 minutes or until set. Center will be slightly soft when it is done.

Per serving (excluding unknown items): 288.7 Calories; 24.8 Fat (77.2 calories from fat); 14.2 Protein; 2.3 Carbohydrate; 171 Cholesterol; 350 Sodium.

Miniature Quiches

Makes 4 servings.

1/2 cup green bell pepper chopped
1/4 cup scallions chopped
2 eggs beaten
2 egg whites beaten
1 teaspoon chili powder
1/2 teaspoon ground cumin
1/8 teaspoon ground red pepper
1/2 cup cheddar cheese shredded

Preheat oven to 425 degrees. Saute bell pepper and scallions until tender. Beat all eggs slightly. Stir in sauteed vegetables with eggs and then all remaining ingredients. Spoon one tablespoon of mix into small muffin tins. Bake until centers are set, about 8 to 10 minutes. Allow to cool a minute and then remove from tin. (They may need a bit of persuasion with a knife around the edges.) Serve hot or warm. Makes around 20 little quiches.

Per serving (excluding unknown items): 106.1 Calories; 7.1 Fat (60.0 calories from fat); 8.3 Protein; 2.3 Carbohydrate; 106 Cholesterol; 151 Sodium.

Broccoli-Sausage Quiche

Makes 4 servings.

1 pound sausage ground
10 ounces frozen broccoli flowerets
1 cup heavy cream
8 ounces processed American cheese
1 cup cheddar cheese grated
4 eggs well beaten
1 cup mozzarella cheese grated

Preheat oven to 350 degrees. Cook sausage and broccoli separate. In double boiler, heat cream, cheddar and processed cheese (Velveeta), until melted. Let cool. Add eggs and mix well. Layer sausage and broccoli and pour egg mixture over all. Sprinkle with Mozzarella. Bake 30 to 45 minutes until nicely browned.

Per serving (excluding unknown items): 1179.6 Calories; 106.3 Fat (80.8 calories from fat); 47.7 Protein; 9.1 Carbohydrate; 451 Cholesterol; 1949 Sodium.

Southwestern Quiche

Makes 4 servings.

8 eggs
1 cup heavy cream
salt and pepper
4 skinless boneless chicken breasts cooked and diced
1 1/2 cups cheddar cheese shredded
4 ounces green chiles diced
1/4 small onion minced

Mix all ingredients well and place in a very good nonstick pie pan. Bake in a 375 degree oven for 30 to 40 minutes.

Per serving (excluding unknown items): 697.4 Calories; 46.8 Fat (61.3 calories from fat); 61.1 Protein; 5.5 Carbohydrate; 589 Cholesterol; 503 Sodium.

Pepperoni Fritata

Makes 6 servings.

1/4 pound pepperoni slices
4 ounces mozzarella cheese shredded
6 eggs
1/2 cup Parmesan cheese grated
2 teaspoons butter
1 medium onion sliced
1/2 cup mushrooms sliced
1 medium green pepper
1 cup broccoli chopped

Place butter in frying pan. Add onion, mushrooms, pepperoni, green pepper and broccoli. Saute for 3 to 4 minutes until onion is almost done. Beat eggs with Parmesan cheese. Pour over vegetables in frying pan. Do not cover. Let cook until eggs are just about cooked, then sprinkle with Mozzarella cheese. Cook until cheese melts and serve.

Per serving (excluding unknown items): 276.7 Calories; 20.6 Fat (67.2 calories from fat); 17.1 Protein; 5.6 Carbohydrate; 224 Cholesterol; 660 Sodium.

Chili Rellenos Quiche

Makes 4 servings.

2 cups Monterey jack cheese grated
4 ounces chili peppers, canned diced
4 eggs
1 cup heavy cream
1/4 teaspoon pepper

You must use a very good non-stick pie pan for this, unless you are making it in a pie shell for the rest of your family.
Sprinkle one cup of Monterey Jack cheese into pie pan. Layer with half of the can of chilies. Sprinkle with other one cup of Monterey Jack cheese. Add more chilies if you like it hot. Mix together eggs, heavy cream and pepper. Pour over mixture in pie pan. Bake in preheated 375 degree oven for 30 minutes.

Per serving (excluding unknown items): 486.1 Calories; 43.3 Fat (79.4 calories from fat); 20.7 Protein; 4.6 Carbohydrate; 315 Cholesterol; 378 Sodium.

Baked Shrimp with Chili-Garlic Butter

Makes 4 servings.

1 1/2 pounds shrimp in shells
1/2 cup butter
1/4 cup vegetable oil
8 cloves garlic finely chopped
2 dried arbol chilies crumbed
1 tablespoon fresh lime juice
1/4 teaspoon salt

Preheat oven to 400 degrees. Shell and devein shrimp, leaving tails attached; rinse and drain well. Heat butter and oil in small skillet over medium heat until butter is melted and foamy. Add garlic, chilies, lime juice and salt. Cook and stir 1 minute. Remove from heat. Arrange shrimp in even layer in shallow 2-quart baking dish. Pour hot butter mixture over shrimp. Bake shrimp 10 to 12 minutes until shrimp turn pink and opaque, stirring once. Do not overcook or shrimp will be dry and tough.

Per serving (excluding unknown items): 510.4 Calories; 39.2 Fat (69.5 calories from fat); 35.2 Protein; 3.7 Carbohydrate; 320 Cholesterol; 618 Sodium.

Louisiana Grilled Shrimp

Makes 4 servings.

1 pound large shrimp
1/2 cup olive oil
1/2 cup fresh lemon juice
1 teaspoon Cajun seasoning
1 tablespoon Worcestershire sauce
2 large bell peppers cut into 2" pieces
1/4 cup butter melted
1 dash Tabasco sauce

Place unpeeled shrimp in 2 quart casserole. Mix together olive oil, lemon juice, Cajun seasoning, and Worcestershire sauce. Drizzle over shrimp and marinate for at least 4 hours. Remove from marinade and skewer with chunks of pepper between shrimp. Mix butter and Tabasco sauce and brush over shrimp. Grill over hot coals until browned.

Per serving (excluding unknown items): 483.3 Calories; 40.4 Fat (74.4 calories from fat); 23.8 Protein; 7.5 Carbohydrate; 203 Cholesterol; 376 Sodium.

Grilled Soft-Shelled Crabs with Mustard Butter

Makes 6 servings.

4 tablespoons unsalted butter
3 tablespoons Dijon mustard
1/2 teaspoon ground pepper
12 soft-shelled crabs, cleaned

Prepare a medium-hot fire in a covered charcoal or gas grill. Oil the grill rack. In a small saucepan, cook the butter over medium-low heat until it melts, just begins to brown and smells nutty. Immediately remove from the heat and whisk in the mustard and pepper. Liberally brush the mustard butter all over the crabs. Grill the crabs, back side down, until lightly browned, about 3 to 5 minutes. Brush with more mustard butter, turn and grill on the other side until lightly browned and cooked through, about 3 to 5 minutes longer. Serve with any remaining mustard butter drizzled on top.

Per serving (excluding unknown items): 77.7 Calories; 8.5 Fat (94.8 calories from fat); 0.5 Protein; 0.6 Carbohydrate; 22 Cholesterol; 95 Sodium.

Shrimp Scampi

Makes 2 servings.

1 pound shrimp
1 1/2 sticks butter
1/2 teaspoon salt
6 cloves garlic
2 tablespoons fresh parsley chopped
1 teaspoon lemon peel grated
1/2 tablespoon lemon juice fresh or frozen

Shell and devein shrimp. Wash and drain. Melt butter in baking dish or skillet. Saute salt, garlic and 1 tablespoon of parsley. Arrange shrimp in a single layer. Preheat oven to 350 degrees. Bake uncover for five minutes. Turn shrimp over, add lemon juice, lemon peel and remaining parsley. Bake another 8 to 10 minutes. Be careful not to overcook. Baste shrimp with butter garlic sauce. Pour remainder in a small bowl for dipping.

Per serving (excluding unknown items): 330.5 Calories; 12.4 Fat (34.8 calories from fat); 46.8 Protein; 5.4 Carbohydrate; 368 Cholesterol; 959 Sodium.

Blackened Red Snapper Fillets

Makes 4 servings.

1 1/2 tablespoons chili powder
1 tablespoon paprika
1 teaspoon salt
1 teaspoon onion powder
1 teaspoon garlic powder
1/2 teaspoon ground cumin
1/2 teaspoon cayenne
1/2 teaspoon ground pepper
4 red snapper fillets

In a small dish, mix together the chili powder, paprika, salt, onion powder, garlic powder, cumin, cayenne and black pepper. Prepare a medium fire in a covered charcoal or gas grill. Oil the grill rack. Sprinkle both sides of the fish with the spice mixture, patting it in lightly with your fingertips. Cover and grill the fish, skin side down, for 4 minutes. Turn and grill until the fish is just opaque throughout, about 4 minutes longer.

Per serving (excluding unknown items): 106.2 Calories; 2.0 Fat (16.8 calories from fat); 18.3 Protein; 3.9 Carbohydrate; 31 Cholesterol; 618 Sodium.

Spanish Baked Fish

Makes 6 servings.

1 1/2 pounds fish fillets
1/2 teaspoon salt
1/4 teaspoon paprika
1/4 teaspoon pepper
1 green pepper cut in rings
1 tomato sliced
1 onion sliced
2 tablespoons lemon juice
2 tablespoons olive oil
1 garlic clove minced
2 lemons

Cut the 2 lemons into wedges.

Cut fish into serving-sized pieces. Place in oven-proof baking dish. Sprinkle with salt, paprika and pepper. Top with green pepper rings, tomato slices and onion slices.

Mix lemon juice, oil and garlic. Pour over the fish fillets. COVER and bake 15 minutes at 375 degrees. UNCOVER and bake about 10-13 minutes longer or until fish flakes easily. Serve with lemon wedges.

Per serving (excluding unknown items): 151.1 Calories; 5.4 Fat (31.5 calories from fat); 20.9 Protein; 5.5 Carbohydrate; 49 Cholesterol; 241 Sodium.

Shrimp On Skewers

Makes 4 servings.

24 large shrimp peeled and deveined
3 cloves garlic minced
3 tablespoons chopped fresh parsley
2 tablespoons chopped fresh oregano
1/2 cup olive oil
1/4 cup brandy or dry white wine
salt and freshly ground pepper to taste
lemon wedges for accompaniment

In a large bowl combine all ingredients except lemon wedges. Mix well and marinate at least 1 hour, or cover and refrigerate up to 4 hours. Preheat broiler. Remove shrimp, reserving marinade; thread 6 shrimp onto each of 4 metal skewers. Place on a broiler rack with a pan underneath to catch drippings. Pour marinade over shrimp. Broil about 3 inches from heat, basting with marinade and turning once, until golden on both sides (about 10 minutes total cooking time).

Per serving (excluding unknown items): 336.2 Calories; 28.4 Fat (78.1 calories from fat); 16.1 Protein; 1.8 Carbohydrate; 119 Cholesterol; 118 Sodium.

Deep Fried Shrimp

Makes 2 servings.

1 pound shrimp shelled, deveined
2 eggs
splash heavy cream
1 package pork skins crushed
salt

Clean and devein shrimp, removing shells but leaving tails attached. Mix eggs with a splash of heavy cream. Dip shrimp into egg mixture and roll in crushed pork skins. Deep fry until browned.

Per serving (excluding unknown items): 310.6 Calories; 8.5 Fat (25.9 calories from fat); 52.1 Protein; 2.6 Carbohydrate; 530 Cholesterol; 417 Sodium.

Grilled Shrimp Espanol

Makes 6 servings.

3/4 cup dry sherry
1/2 cup olive oil
3 tablespoons lemon juice
8 cloves garlic crushed
1/2 teaspoon ground pepper
1/8 teaspoon cayenne
1 1/2 pounds large shrimp shelled, deveined

In a shallow dish just large enough to hold the shrimp, combine the sherry, olive oil, lemon juice, garlic, pepper and cayenne. Add the shrimp and turn to coat completely. Let stand for 30 minutes. Prepare a hot fire in a covered charcoal or gas grill. Thread the shrimp onto single or double skewers. Pour the marinade into a small saucepan and boil 3 minutes. Grill the shrimp, turning once, until they are pink and firm to the touch, about 4 to 6 minutes total. Slide the shrimp off the skewers onto a platter. Pour the sauce over the shrimp.

Per serving (excluding unknown items): 321.3 Calories; 20.0 Fat (62.7 calories from fat); 23.4 Protein; 3.4 Carbohydrate; 173 Cholesterol; 172 Sodium.

Foiled Fish on the Grill

Makes 4 servings.

1 pound fish fillets
2 tablespoons margarine not diet
1/4 cup lemon juice
1 tablespoon fresh parsley chopped
1 teaspoon fresh dill weed
1 teaspoon salt
1/4 teaspoon black pepper
1/4 teaspoon paprika
1 onion thinly sliced

Use heavy aluminum foil cut into large squares. Place equal portions of the fish fillets on each piece of foil.

In a saucepan, melt margarine. Add lemon juice, parsley, dill, salt and pepper. Stir to blend well. Pour this mixture over the fish, sprinkle with paprika, and top with the onion slices which have been separated into rings. Fold the foil around the mixture and sea tightly. Leave a little space for the food to expand while cooking.

Place on hot grill and grill for 5-7 minutes per side. Fish should flake easily when done.

Per serving (excluding unknown items): 162.7 Calories; 6.5 Fat (36.4 calories from fat); 20.8 Protein; 4.8 Carbohydrate; 49 Cholesterol; 663 Sodium.

Vegetables

Green Beans Picante

Makes 4 servings.

1 tablespoon butter
1/4 small onion sliced into rings
16 ounces green beans, canned drained
1/4 cup picante sauce
1/4 teaspoon salt
1/4 teaspoon pepper
1/4 teaspoon lemon juice

In saucepan melt butter and saute onions until tender. Add green beans, picante sauce, salt, pepper and lemon juice. Cover and heat thoroughly.

Per serving (excluding unknown items): 50.5 Calories; 3.2 Fat (50.4 calories from fat); 1.3 Protein; 5.9 Carbohydrate; 8 Cholesterol; 556 Sodium.

Cheddar Squash Bake

Makes 8 servings.

6 cups squash thinly sliced
2 egg yolks slightly beaten
1 cup sour cream
2 tablespoons flour
2 egg whites stiffly beaten
1 1/2 cups cheddar cheese shredded
6 slices bacon cooked

Steam cook squash. Mix next three ingredients. Fold in whites. Layer half the squash, egg mixture and cheese in baking dish. Crumble bacon and sprinkle on top. Repeat layers.

Per serving (excluding unknown items): 219.2 Calories; 16.9 Fat (68.2 calories from fat); 10.5 Protein; 7.2 Carbohydrate; 92 Cholesterol; 240 Sodium.

Blushing Cauliflower

Makes 6 servings.

1 head cauliflower
1/2 teaspoon salt
2 tablespoons butter
1 clove garlic crushed
10 ounces tomato soup, condensed
1/2 cup American cheese grated

Place cauliflower in a large pan. Add salted water to cover bottom of the pan. Simmer over low heat for about 20 to 30 minutes, or until tender. Melt butter in a saucepan. Saute garlic until lightly browned. Add soup and cheese. Heat, stirring occasionally, over low heat until cheese is melted. Pour sauce over cauliflower.

Per serving (excluding unknown items): 103.3 Calories; 7.5 Fat (62.8 calories from fat); 3.1 Protein; 6.9 Carbohydrate; 19 Cholesterol; 608 Sodium.

Herb Buttered Zucchini Fans

Makes 4 servings.

1/3 cup butter softened
2 tablespoons parsley minced
1/2 teaspoon dried tarragon
1/8 teaspoon salt
1/8 teaspoon pepper
4 small zucchini
1/4 cup water
2 tablespoons parmesan cheese freshly grated

Combine first five ingredients and set aside. Cut each zucchini into lengthwise slices, leaving slices attached on stem end. Fan slices out and spread evenly with butter mixture. Place in a 15-x-10-1 inch pan; add water. Bake at 400 degrees for 20 minutes or until crisp-tender. Sprinkle cheese on zucchini and broil four inches from heat for two minutes or until cheese melts.

Per serving (excluding unknown items): 168.4 Calories; 16.1 Fat (82.2 calories from fat); 3.1 Protein; 4.8 Carbohydrate; 43 Cholesterol; 280 Sodium.

Country Cabbage

Makes 6 servings.

1 onion chopped
1 1/2 tablespoons butter
1 cabbage cut into wedges
1 tomato chopped
salt and pepper

Saute onions in butter until tender. Add cabbage and tomato. Sprinkle with salt and pepper. Cover and cook over low heat for 20 to 30 minutes or until cabbage is tender.

Per serving (excluding unknown items): 55.5 Calories; 3.1 Fat (45.9 calories from fat); 1.9 Protein; 6.3 Carbohydrate; 8 Cholesterol; 53 Sodium.

Baked Eggplant Napoli

Makes 8 servings.

1/2 cup onion chopped
2 tablespoons oil
10 ounces tomato puree
2/3 cup water
1 1/2 teaspoons salt
1 teaspoon oregano
dash pepper
1 medium eggplant peeled and sliced
2 cups cheddar cheese grated

In a skillet saute chopped onions in oil. Add tomato puree, water, salt, oregano and pepper. Bring to a boil and simmer for 15 minutes.
In a greased 2-quart baking dish, alternate layers of sliced eggplant, tomato sauce and 1 cup grated cheese, starting with layer of eggplant and ending with layer of tomato sauce. Bake at 350 degrees for one hour. A few minutes before removing from oven, sprinkle remaining cheese over top and continue heating until cheese melts.

Per serving (excluding unknown items): 175.2 Calories; 13.0 Fat (64.6 calories from fat); 8.3 Protein; 7.7 Carbohydrate; 30 Cholesterol; 719 Sodium.

Zucchini Parmesan

Makes 10 servings.

1/4 cup peanut oil
8 medium zucchini thinly sliced
1/4 cup onion chopped
2 tablespoons parsley chopped
1 clove garlic minced
1 tablespoon salt
1/4 teaspoon pepper
1/4 teaspoon oregano
1/4 teaspoon rosemary
2 cups tomatoes peeled and chopped
1/2 cup Parmesan cheese grated

Heat peanut oil in large skillet. Add zucchini, onion, parsley, garlic, salt, pepper, oregano and rosemary. Saute mixture over medium heat, stirring often, until zucchini is tender, about 20 minutes. Toss in tomatoes and continue to saute until tomatoes are thoroughly heated, about five minutes. Turn mixture into a serving dish. Sprinkle with Parmesan cheese.

Per serving (excluding unknown items): 94.6 Calories; 6.8 Fat (61.0 calories from fat); 3.4 Protein; 6.4 Carbohydrate; 3 Cholesterol; 724 Sodium.

Cool 'N Creamy Coleslaw

Makes 10 servings.

2 envelopes gelatin powder, unsweetened
2 packets Sweet 'n Low® sweetener
1 3/4 cups boiling water
1 1/3 cups mayonnaise
1/4 cup lemon juice
4 cups cabbage shredded
1 cup carrots shredded
1/4 cup onion finely chopped

In large bowl, mix unflavored gelatine and sweetener. Add boiling water and stir until gelatin is completely dissolved. Blend in mayonnaise and lemon juice. Chill until mixture is consistency of unbeaten egg whites. Stir in cabbage, carrots and onion. Pour into 11x7-inch pan and chill until firm. To serve, cut into squares.

Per serving (excluding unknown items): 253.6 Calories; 25.0 Fat (82.9 calories from fat); 8.8 Protein; 2.8 Carbohydrate; 10 Cholesterol; 185 Sodium.

Grilled Jack Cheese-Stuffed Peppers

Makes 6 servings.

6 poblano peppers
1 tablespoon vegetable oil
4 ounces Monterey jack cheese

Prepare grill with a medium-hot fire. Brush the peppers with half of the oil and grill, turning often, until the skins are blackened and the peppers are tender, about 10 to 12 minutes. Peel away the blackened skin from the peppers and cut a small slit in the stem end. Insert a small knife and scrape off as many of the seeds as possible. Shake out the seeds. Cut the cheese into 6 rectangular sticks or pieces small enough to fit into the slit in the peppers. Insert the cheese in the peppers, taking care not to break the peppers. (If the peppers should split, simply wrap them around the cheese and secure with wet toothpicks.) Brush the peppers with the remaining oil. Grill, turning once with a spatula, until the peppers are tinged with brown and the cheese is melted, about 3 to 5 minutes.

Per serving (excluding unknown items): 108.1 Calories; 8.1 Fat (65.0 calories from fat); 5.5 Protein; 4.3 Carbohydrate; 17 Cholesterol; 104 Sodium.

Spinach-Stuffed Squash

Makes 6 servings.

3 medium yellow squash
1/4 cup butter
1 tablespoon flour
1/2 cup whipping cream
1/2 teaspoon salt
1/8 teaspoon ground nutmeg
1 package frozen spinach chopped, thawed

Steam squash 8 to 10 minutes or until tender. Cut squash in half lengthwise; scoop out pulp, leaving shells intact. Keep warm.
Melt butter in a heavy saucepan over low heat; add flour, stirring until smooth. Cook one minute, stirring constantly. Gradually add whipping cream; cook over medium heat, stirring constantly, until thickened and bubbly. Stir in salt and nutmeg. Stir spinach into creamed mixture and cook until thoroughly heated. Spoon mixture into shells. Serve immediately.

Per serving (excluding unknown items): 170.8 Calories; 15.3 Fat (76.1 calories from fat); 3.6 Protein; 7.3 Carbohydrate; 48 Cholesterol; 320 Sodium.

Broccoli Casserole

Makes 8 servings.

16 ounces broccoli, frozen chopped
2 cups American cheese grated
1 can cream of mushroom soup, condensed

Cook frozen broccoli according to directions on package. Drain broccoli and add cream of mushroom soup and one cup of grated cheese. Pour into a greased casserole and top with remaining one cup of cheese. Bake in 350 degree oven until hot and cheese is melted.

Per serving (excluding unknown items): 160.4 Calories; 11.9 Fat (64.9 calories from fat); 8.5 Protein; 6.0 Carbohydrate; 27 Cholesterol; 507 Sodium.

Tex-Mex Coleslaw

Makes 12 servings.

3 small avocados mashed
2 tablespoons lemon juice
6 cups cabbage shredded
1 cup onion finely chopped
1/2 cup mayonnaise
1 1/2 packets Sweet 'n Low® sweetener
1 tablespoon tarragon vinegar
1/2 teaspoon salt
1/4 teaspoon garlic powder
1/4 teaspoon pepper
dash hot sauce
dash Worcestershire sauce

Combine avocados and lemon juice in a large bowl, mixing well. Add shredded cabbage and chopped onion. Mix well. Combine mayonnaise, sweetener, vinegar, salt, garlic powder, pepper, hot sauce and Worcestershire. Stir into mixture.

Per serving (excluding unknown items): 137.1 Calories; 13.6 Fat (82.0 calories from fat); 1.4 Protein; 5.3 Carbohydrate; 3 Cholesterol; 151 Sodium.

Summer Squash Casserole

Makes 6 servings.

1 pound yellow squash cut in 1" pieces
1/4 cup mayonnaise
1 egg beaten
1 cup cheddar cheese shredded
2 tablespoons butter
1/2 cup onion chopped

Steam squash in small amount of water until tender and drain. Meanwhile, mix together mayonnaise, egg, 1/2 cup of cheese, two tablespoons of melted butter and onion. Add the squash and place in round casserole dish. Sprinkle remaining cheese over top of squash and bake in 350 degree oven until cheese is melted.

Per serving (excluding unknown items): 205.3 Calories; 18.7 Fat (78.8 calories from fat); 6.7 Protein; 4.6 Carbohydrate; 63 Cholesterol; 219 Sodium.

Creamed Spinach

Makes 8 servings.

2 packages spinach cooked and drained
1/3 cup sour cream
1/4 teaspoon salt
1/8 teaspoon ground nutmeg
dash of pepper

Cook frozen spinach as directed. Drain. Stir in remaining ingredients and heat through.

Per serving (excluding unknown items): 22.9 Calories; 2.1 Fat (77.4 calories from fat); 0.6 Protein; 0.8 Carbohydrate; 4 Cholesterol; 80 Sodium.

Elegant Puffed Broccoli

Makes 8 servings.

2 bunches broccoli cut into spears
2 egg whites at room temperature
1/4 teaspoon salt
1/2 cup Swiss cheese shredded
1/2 cup mayonnaise

Arrange hot cooked broccoli in shallow 1-1/2 quart pan or broiler proof serving dish. In small bowl with mixer at high speed beat egg whites and salt until stiff peaks form. Fold in cheese and mayonnaise; spoon evenly over broccoli. Broil six inches from source of heat four minutes or until golden brown. Serve immediately.

Per serving (excluding unknown items): 135.5 Calories; 13.7 Fat (85.7 calories from fat); 3.7 Protein; 1.5 Carbohydrate; 11 Cholesterol; 183 Sodium.

Italian Green Beans

Makes 6 servings.

1 pound green beans
1 teaspoon olive oil
1 clove garlic minced
1/2 cup red bell pepper sliced thin
2 tablespoons water
2 tablespoons butter
salt and pepper

Steam green beans in small amount of water until tender. Drain. In skillet, saute garlic in the olive oil. Add the red peppers and green beans. Saute an additional three to four minutes. Add two tablespoons of water. Cover and simmer to desired consistency. Add butter. Salt and pepper to taste.

Per serving (excluding unknown items): 63.6 Calories; 4.6 Fat (60.6 calories from fat); 1.3 Protein; 5.4 Carbohydrate; 10 Cholesterol; 43 Sodium.

Broth-Simmered Brussels Sprouts

Makes 6 servings.

1 pound Brussels sprouts
1/2 cup beef broth
1 tablespoon butter softened
1/4 cup grated Parmesan cheese
paprika

Use large enough saucepan to allow sprouts to fit in single layer. Pour broth into saucepan. Place sprouts, stem ends down, in broth. Bring to a boil over high heat. Reduce heat to medium-low. Cover and simmer about 5 minutes or just until sprouts turn bright green and are crisp-tender when pierced with fork. Uncover. Simmer until liquid is almost evaporated. Toss cooked sprouts with butter, then cheese. Transfer to serving dish and sprinkle with paprika to taste.

Per serving (excluding unknown items): 39.2 Calories; 3.4 Fat (77.7 calories from fat); 1.9 Protein; 0.3 Carbohydrate; 9 Cholesterol; 228 Sodium.

Spinach Casserole

Makes 8 servings.

10 ounces frozen spinach chopped
2 tablespoons flour
1/4 cup butter melted
1 pint cottage cheese small curd
3 eggs slightly beaten
1/2 cup cheddar cheese shredded

Preheat oven to 350 degrees. Grease a 1-1/2 quart casserole dish. Mix all ingredients together. Place in the baking dish and bake for 50 to 60 minutes.

Per serving (excluding unknown items): 168.7 Calories; 10.8 Fat (57.5 calories from fat); 12.8 Protein; 5.2 Carbohydrate; 96 Cholesterol; 378 Sodium.

Cauliflower-Cheese Casserole

Makes 4 servings.

1 small cauliflower
1 cup heavy cream
2 cups cheddar cheese shredded
1 egg
1/3 cup onion sauted

Steam cauliflower until tender. Chop into small pieces and place in the bottom of a baking dish. Combine remaining ingredients. Pour over cauliflower and bake at 350 degrees for 45 minutes.

Per serving (excluding unknown items): 456.7 Calories; 41.9 Fat (81.7 calories from fat); 17.0 Protein; 4.2 Carbohydrate; 186 Cholesterol; 391 Sodium.

Stuffed Squash Mexican

Makes 6 servings.

3 medium yellow squash (1 pound)
2 cloves garlic chopped
1/4 cup onion chopped
1/4 cup green pepper chopped
1 jalapeno seeded and chopped
1 tablespoon olive oil
1 teaspoon chili powder
1/4 teaspoon salt and pepper each
3/4 cup Monterey jack cheese shredded
3 tablespoons sour cream
2 tablespoons picante sauce

Cook squash in boiling water until tender but still firm. Drain and cool slightly. Remove and discard stems. Cut each squash in half lengthwise; scoop out pulp, leaving a 1/4-inch shell. Reserve the pulp. Saute garlic, onion, green pepper and jalapeno in olive oil until crisp-tender. Stir in squash pulp and cook, stirring often, until liquid has been absorbed. Add chili powder, salt and pepper; remove from heat. Add Monterey Jack cheese and sour cream; stir mixture well. Place squash shells in a lightly greased baking dish. Spoon squash mixture evenly into shells. Bake at 350 degrees for 25 minutes. Divide picante sauce among squash; bake an additional five minutes.

Per serving (excluding unknown items): 109.7 Calories; 8.3 Fat (65.1 calories from fat); 4.8 Protein; 5.3 Carbohydrate; 16 Cholesterol; 181 Sodium.

Green Bean Bundles

Makes 8 servings.

2 cans green beans whole
1/3 cup Sugar Twin brown sugar
1/3 cup margarine melted
dash garlic salt
4 slices bacon

Drain two cans of green beans. Divide into individual servings and wrap with 1/2 slice of uncooked bacon. Place in a baking dish. Mix together brown sugar, melted margarine and garlic salt. Pour over green beans. Bake in 350 degree oven for 30 minutes.

Per serving (excluding unknown items): 93.3 Calories; 9.1 Fat (86.2 calories from fat); 1.5 Protein; 1.8 Carbohydrate; 3 Cholesterol; 141 Sodium.

Cauliflower Souffle

Makes 2 servings.

1 cup cauliflower steamed and mashed
2 eggs
1/2 cup cottage cheese
4 tablespoons cheddar cheese grated
salt and pepper

Mix all ingredients together. Place in casserole dish. Bake in 350 degree oven for 20 minutes.

Per serving (excluding unknown items): 175.9 Calories; 10.1 Fat (52.2 calories from fat); 17.0 Protein; 3.8 Carbohydrate; 203 Cholesterol; 377 Sodium.

Sour Cream Cucumbers

Makes 8 servings.

1/2 cup white vinegar
1/2 cup water
1 packet Sweet 'n Low® sweetener
1/2 teaspoon salt
2 medium cucumbers cut into 1/8" slices
1/2 cup sour cream
1/2 teaspoon white pepper

Mix vinegar, water, sugar and salt. Pour over cucumbers in glass or plastic bowl. Cover and refrigerate at least two but not longer than 24 hours; drain. Mix in sour cream and pepper. Serve immediately.

Per serving (excluding unknown items): 52.8 Calories; 3.2 Fat (50.1 calories from fat); 1.5 Protein; 5.7 Carbohydrate; 6 Cholesterol; 145 Sodium.

Country Fried Okra

Makes 4 servings.

2 cups okra cut in 1/2" slices
2 eggs
1 tablespoon heavy cream
1 cup pork skins crushed

Beat eggs with a splash of heavy cream. Place crushed pork skins in a plastic container. Dip okra into egg mixture. Add the dipped okra to the pork skins. Place lid on container and shake until okra is well covered. Fry in 1/2-inch of hot oil. When brown and crispy, remove with slotted spoon and drain on paper towels.

Per serving (excluding unknown items): 116.4 Calories; 7.0 Fat (55.3 calories from fat); 9.1 Protein; 3.6 Carbohydrate; 111 Cholesterol; 261 Sodium.

Spinach Souffle

Makes 8 servings.

4 tablespoons flour
3 eggs
1 package spinach, frozen thawed and drained
1/2 pound cottage cheese
1/2 pound cheddar cheese grated
1/2 teaspoon salt

Beat together flour and eggs until smooth. Add one package of spinach, cottage cheese, cheddar cheese and salt. Place in a greased 8x8x2-inch baking dish. Bake in a preheated 350 degree oven for one hour or until slightly browned. Let set a few minutes before cutting.

Per serving (excluding unknown items): 182.3 Calories; 11.6 Fat (57.6 calories from fat); 13.9 Protein; 5.3 Carbohydrate; 101 Cholesterol; 459 Sodium.

Baked Broccoli and Cheese

Makes 6 servings.

3 medium fresh broccoli
6 eggs
6 tablespoons soy flour
1/4 cup margarine
8 ounces American cheese grated
12 ounces cottage cheese

Cook broccoli in salt water until tender. Drain. Mix eggs, soy flour, butter and both cheeses together in a bowl. Add drained broccoli. Mix. Pour into glass baking dish and bake in a 350 degree oven for 45 minutes. The dish should be greased on sides and bottom before putting mixture in.

Per serving (excluding unknown items): 359.1 Calories; 26.0 Fat (64.5 calories from fat); 24.7 Protein; 7.4 Carbohydrate; 224 Cholesterol; 631 Sodium.

Company Cauliflower

Makes 4 servings.

1 medium cauliflower
1 cup mayonnaise
1 tablespoon prepared mustard
1 teaspoon dried mustard
4 ounces sharp cheddar cheese shredded

Place whole head of cauliflower, stem end down, in and 8" glass pie plate. Cover with plastic wrap. Microwave on high 7 to 8 minutes or until tender. Mix mayonnaise, prepared mustard and dry mustard in a bowl. Pour mayonnaise mixture over top of cooked cauliflower. Sprinkle with shredded cheese. Microwave on high one minute to melt cheese.

Per serving (excluding unknown items): 513.6 Calories; 56.3 Fat (93.3 calories from fat); 8.0 Protein; 1.1 Carbohydrate; 49 Cholesterol; 538 Sodium.

Squash Casserole

Makes 8 servings.

2 pounds yellow squash
1 small onion
2 eggs beaten
2 tablespoons butter
salt and pepper to taste
2 tablespoons margarine
2 tablespoons flour
1/2 cup heavy cream
1/2 cup water
1/2 teaspoon salt
1 cup cheddar cheese grated

White sauce: Melt margarine, stir in flour until smooth. Add salt, cream and water. Cook, stirring constantly, until it thickens. Add cheese. Cook squash and onion in small amount of water until done. Drain any remaining water. Add beaten eggs, melted butter, salt and pepper. Add white sauce mixed with cheese; mix well. Pour into greased casserole. Cheese may be sprinkled on top. Bake at 350 degrees until hot.

Per serving (excluding unknown items): 210.3 Calories; 17.2 Fat (71.5 calories from fat); 6.9 Protein; 8.5 Carbohydrate; 89 Cholesterol; 306 Sodium.

Desserts

Creamy Chocolate Pie

Makes 8 servings.

1 Pecan Pie Crust (see recipe)
1 package Jell-O Sugar Free Chocolate Pudding
1 cup heavy cream
1/2 cup water
8 ounces cream cheese

Mix together pudding with heavy cream and water. Blend in cream cheese until smooth. Pour pudding batter into Pecan Pie Crust shell. Refrigerate until well chilled.

Per serving (excluding unknown items): 230.3 Calories; 22.3 Fat (82.7 calories from fat); 3.4 Protein; 7.2 Carbohydrate; 73 Cholesterol; 156 Sodium.

Strawberry-Banana Cream

Makes 6 servings.

1 cup water
1 teaspoon banana extract
1 package Sugar-Free Strawberry-Banana Jello
2 tablespoons No-cal Strawberry Syrup
1/2 cup Diet Strawberry Soda
6 tablespoons heavy cream

Heat water to a boil. Add extract. Pour over Jello and completely dissolve it. Add syrup, soda and cream. Whisk until well blended. Refrigerate until firm.

Per serving (excluding unknown items): 51.3 Calories; 5.5 Fat (94.5 calories from fat); 0.3 Protein; 0.4 Carbohydrate; 20 Cholesterol; 7 Sodium.

Chocolate Cheesecake

Makes 8 servings.

16 ounces cream cheese
3 egg
1 cup sour cream
1 tablespoon vanilla extract
15 packets Sweet 'n Low® sweetener
1 package Jell-O Sugar Free Chocolate Pudding

Preheat oven to 350 degrees. Place all ingredients in bowl and blend for 15 minutes. Pour mixture into 9-inch non-stick pie pan. Bake one hour. After baking one hour, turn oven off and leave cake in oven for an additional one hour. Refrigerate.

Per serving (excluding unknown items): 311.0 Calories; 27.4 Fat (79.1 calories from fat); 7.7 Protein; 8.6 Carbohydrate; 143 Cholesterol; 265 Sodium.

Cinnamon Toasted Nuts

Makes 4 servings.

1 teaspoon butter
1/2 cup pecans
2 packages Sweet 'n Low® sweetener
1 tablespoon cinnamon

Melt butter in non-stick pan. Stir in nuts and saute until lightly browned. Sprinkle with sugar/cinnamon.

Per serving (excluding unknown items): 62.5 Calories; 5.8 Fat (77.9 calories from fat); 0.6 Protein; 3.1 Carbohydrate; 3 Cholesterol; 12 Sodium.

Baked Custard

Makes 6 servings.

3 eggs slightly beaten
8 packets Sweet 'n Low® sweetener
2 cups heavy cream
1/2 teaspoon vanilla

Heat cream in saucepan. Combine eggs, sugar and 1/4 teaspoon of salt. Slowly stir in lightly cooled cream and vanilla. Fill six 6-ounce custard cups; set in shallow pan on oven rack. Pour hot water into pan one inch deep. Bake at 325 degrees for 40 to 45 minutes or until knife comes out clean. Serve warm or chilled. To unmold chilled, first loosen edges then slip point of knife down the side to let air in. Invert.

Per serving (excluding unknown items): 311.7 Calories; 31.5 Fat (89.8 calories from fat); 4.3 Protein; 3.8 Carbohydrate; 200 Cholesterol; 62 Sodium.

Cloud Nine Pie

Makes 8 servings.

1 Pecan Pie Crust (see recipe)
8 ounces cream cheese
8 packets Sweet 'n Low® sweetener
1 cup heavy cream
1 tablespoon vanilla extract
2 packets Sweet 'n Low® sweetener
1 tablespoon vanilla

Mix cream cheese and 8 packets of sweetener with electric mixer until well blended. Prepare whipped cream using cream, vanilla, 2 packets of sweetener and 1 tablespoon of vanilla. Gently stir whipped cream into cream cheese. Blend for one minute with electric mixer. Spoon into crust.

Per serving (excluding unknown items): 230.8 Calories; 22.3 Fat (85.2 calories from fat); 2.9 Protein; 5.9 Carbohydrate; 73 Cholesterol; 105 Sodium.

Vanilla Cream Pudding

Makes 4 servings.

12 packets Sweet 'n Low® sweetener
2 tablespoons cornstarch
1/8 teaspoon salt
1 cup heavy cream
1 cup water
2 egg yolks slightly beaten
2 tablespoons butter softened
2 teaspoons vanilla

Mix sweetener, cornstarch and salt in 2-quart saucepan. Stir in cream and water gradually. Cook over medium heat, stirring constantly, until mixture thickens and boils. Boil and stir one minute. Stir at least half of the hot mixture gradually into egg yolks. Stir into hot mixture in saucepan. Boil and stir one minute. Remove from heat. Stir in butter and vanilla. Pour into dessert dishes. Serve warm or cool.

Per serving (excluding unknown items): 319.3 Calories; 30.3 Fat (85.5 calories from fat); 2.7 Protein; 8.9 Carbohydrate; 203 Cholesterol; 165 Sodium.

Peanut Butter Kisses

Makes 12 servings.

2 egg whites
1/8 teaspoon cream of tartar
16 packets Sweet 'n Low® sweetener
1/2 cup peanut butter

In a small bowl with mixer at high speed, beat egg whites and cream of tartar until mixture holds stiff peaks when beater is raised. Add sweetener two packets at a time, beating well after each addition. Continue beating until mixture holds very stiff peaks when beater is raised. Lightly fold in peanut butter just until mixed. Drop by teaspoonfuls onto greased cookie sheet. Bake in 300 degree oven for 25 minutes or until lightly browned. Remove from cookie sheet immediately. Makes about 3 dozen cookies.

Per serving (excluding unknown items): 71.4 Calories; 5.4 Fat (64.3 calories from fat); 3.2 Protein; 3.5 Carbohydrate; 0 Cholesterol; 66 Sodium.

Chocolate Mousse

Makes 6 servings.

2 teaspoons Hershey's® cocoa
4 packages Sweet 'n Low® sweetener
1 teaspoon vanilla
1 pint whipping cream

Pour whipping cream into a bowl. Add the rest of the ingredients and mix with a hand mixer until thickened.

Per serving (excluding unknown items): 279.6 Calories; 29.4 Fat (92.9 calories from fat); 1.7 Protein; 3.4 Carbohydrate; 109 Cholesterol; 33 Sodium.

Pecan Pie Crust

Makes 8 servings.

1 1/2 cups pecan halves ground
3 tablespoons butter melted
2 packets Sweet 'n Low® sweetener

Ground pecan halves with food processor until powder consistency. Combine ground nuts, melted margarine and sugar. Press evenly into bottom and on sides of 9-inch pie plate. Bake at 350 degrees for 10 to 12 minutes. Cool and fill as desired.

Per serving (excluding unknown items): 110.2 Calories; 11.5 Fat (89.5 calories from fat); 0.9 Protein; 2.2 Carbohydrate; 11 Cholesterol; 44 Sodium.

Pumpkin Pie

Makes 8 servings.

4 ounces cream cheese softened
1 tablespoon cream
2 packages Sweet 'n Low® sweetener
1 cup heavy cream whipped
1 Pecan Pie Crust
16 ounces pumpkin
1 package Jell-O Sugar Free Vanilla Pudding
1 teaspoon ground cinnamon
1/2 teaspoon ground ginger
1/4 teaspoon ground cloves

In a large bowl, mix cream cheese, 1 tablespoon of heavy cream and sugar with wire whisk until smooth. Gently stir in 1 1/2 cups prepared whipped cream. Spread on bottom of Pecan Pie Crust. In a second bowl, stir pumpkin, pudding mix and spices into 1/2 cup of heavy cream and 1/2 cup of water. Beat with wire whisk until well blended. (Mixture will be thick.) Spread over cream cheese layer. Refrigerate four hours.

Per serving (excluding unknown items): 198.0 Calories; 17.9 Fat (76.7 calories from fat); 2.3 Protein; 10.0 Carbohydrate; 59 Cholesterol; 61 Sodium.

Mexican Hot Chocolate

Makes 6 servings.

1 cup heavy cream
2 cups water
6 packets Sweet 'n Low® sweetener
1 unsweetened baking chocolate squares crumbled
1/2 teaspoon ground cinnamon
1 egg beaten
1 teaspoon vanilla
whipped cream, pressurized

Combine heavy cream and water. In a large saucepan heat 1/2 cup of the cream mixture, the sweetener, chocolate and cinnamon. Cook and stir over medium-low heat until chocolate is completely melted. Gradually stir in remaining cream. Cook and stir until milk is very hot, but do not boil.
Gradually stir one cup of the hot milk mixture into egg, then transfer entire mixture into saucepan. Cook and stir for two minutes over low heat. Remove from heat and stir in vanilla. Beat with a rotary-type beater until very frothy.
Pour hot chocolate into mugs and dollop with whipped cream.

Per serving (excluding unknown items): 178.8 Calories; 18.0 Fat (87.1 calories from fat); 2.2 Protein; 3.8 Carbohydrate; 84 Cholesterol; 31 Sodium.

No-Bake Chocolate Cheesecake

Makes 8 servings.

1 package unflavored gelatin
1 cup boiling water
16 ounces cream cheese cut in small cubes
1 teaspoon vanilla
18 packages Sweet 'n Low® sweetener
1/2 package Jell-O Sugar Free Chocolate Pudding

In a large bowl, dissolve gelatin in boiling water. Add the cut up cream cheese and whisk until melted. Add the pudding, sweetener and vanilla. Beat with a mixer until thick and creamy. Pour into an 8' pie tin sprayed with Pam. Refrigerate.

Per serving (excluding unknown items): 235.8 Calories; 19.8 Fat (74.8 calories from fat); 9.6 Protein; 5.5 Carbohydrate; 62 Cholesterol; 210 Sodium.

Sweet Cheese

Makes 4 servings.

8 ounces cream cheese
1 egg yolk
6 packets Sweet 'n Low® sweetener
1 tablespoon Jell-O Sugar Free Chocolate Pudding
2 tablespoons Cool Whip®

Cream cheese and yolk. Add sugar and pudding. Either drop by rounded spoonfuls or place in cookie decorator and shape into candies.

Per serving (excluding unknown items): 228.1 Calories; 21.6 Fat (84.1 calories from fat); 5.1 Protein; 4.1 Carbohydrate; 115 Cholesterol; 187 Sodium.

Strawberry Cream

Makes 10 servings.

1 package strawberry gelatin, sugar-free
1 cup boiling water
8 ounces cream cheese
16 packets Sweet 'n Low® sweetener
2 cups whipping cream

Pour boiling water over gelatin, stirring until it dissolves. Add cream cheese, sweetener and whipping cream. Refrigerate until set.

Per serving (excluding unknown items): 252.9 Calories; 25.5 Fat (90.5 calories from fat); 2.7 Protein; 3.4 Carbohydrate; 90 Cholesterol; 92 Sodium.

Vanilla Macadamia Cheesepie

Makes 10 servings.

1 Macadamia Pie Shell
12 ounces cream cheese
1 egg
3/4 cup plain yogurt
10 packages Sweet 'n Low® sweetener
1 tablespoon vanilla

Preheat oven to 350 degrees. Prepare Macadamia Pie Shell. Combine cream cheese, egg, yogurt, sugar and vanilla in medium bowl. Blend thoroughly. Pour cream cheese mixture over crust. Bake 20 minutes or until just set. Cool completely on wire rack. Refrigerate at least two hours.

Per serving (excluding unknown items): 159.5 Calories; 14.2 Fat (72.6 calories from fat); 3.8 Protein; 8.3 Carbohydrate; 60 Cholesterol; 133 Sodium.

Macadamia Pie Shell

Makes 8 servings.

8 squares graham crackers
1 cup macadamia nuts
6 tablespoons butter melted
3 packages Sweet 'n Low® sweetener

Break graham crackers into large pieces. Place in food processor or blender container. Add nuts. Process until finely crushed. Measure 1-3/4 cups. Combine crumb mixture, butter and sugar in small bowl. Press firmly onto bottom and up side of 8-inch pie plate. Refrigerate until firm.

Per serving (excluding unknown items): 142.8 Calories; 13.1 Fat (79.8 calories from fat); 1.0 Protein; 6.4 Carbohydrate; 23 Cholesterol; 131 Sodium.

Popcicles

Makes 12 servings.

1 1/2 cups sugar-free cherry soda
6 tablespoons heavy cream
1 package Sweet 'n Low® sweetener

Mix all ingredients together. Fill plastic popcicle molds and freeze.

Per serving (excluding unknown items): 26.0 Calories; 2.7 Fat (93.6 calories from fat); 0.1 Protein; 0.3 Carbohydrate; 10 Cholesterol; 3 Sodium.

Creamy Fudge

Makes 20 servings.

16 ounces cream cheese softened
2 squares unsweetened baking chocolate melted
12 packets Sweet 'n Low® sweetener
1 teaspoon vanilla extract
1/2 cup pecans chopped

Beat cream cheese, sweetener, chocolate and vanilla until smooth. Stir in pecans. Pour into 8-inch square baking dish that has been lined with foil. Refrigerate overnight. Cut into 20 squares.

Per serving (excluding unknown items): 106.6 Calories; 10.4 Fat (84.3 calories from fat); 2.1 Protein; 2.3 Carbohydrate; 25 Cholesterol; 70 Sodium.

Cheesecake

Makes 8 servings.

40 ounces cream cheese
5 large eggs
2 egg yolks
1/4 cup heavy cream
1/2 teaspoon lemon extract
1/2 teaspoon vanilla extract
36 packets Sweet 'n Low® sweetener

Preheat oven to 475 degrees. Beat cream cheese and sweetener until smooth. Add eggs, egg yolks, heavy cream and both extracts. Beat for an additional five minutes. Pour into a greased springform pan and bake for 12 minutes. Turn oven down to 300 degrees. Bake for 35 minutes longer. Turn oven off but leave cake in for another 30 minutes. Remove and cool completely in pan. Refrigerate overnight.

Per serving (excluding unknown items): 594.0 Calories; 56.1 Fat (84.4 calories from fat); 14.9 Protein; 8.5 Carbohydrate; 333 Cholesterol; 475 Sodium.

Creamy Jello

Makes 12 servings.

3 envelopes sugar-free Jello
3 cups hot water
2 cups sour cream
8 ounces cream cheese

Add sugar-free jello to hot water. Cut cream cheese into small cubes and add to hot water. Whisk until cream cheese is melted. Add sour cream and whisk until smooth. Refrigerate until set.

Per serving (excluding unknown items): 148.1 Calories; 14.6 Fat (87.3 calories from fat); 2.6 Protein; 2.1 Carbohydrate; 38 Cholesterol; 78 Sodium.

Sugared Pecans

Makes 6 servings.

1 egg white
1/4 teaspoon cinnamon
1/2 cup Sugar Twin Brown Sugar
pinch salt
3/4 cup pecan halves

Beat egg white and cinnamon until stiff. Add and continue beating until very stiff brown sugar and pinch of salt. Fold in pecan halves. Drop pecan halves, one at a time, onto a buttered cookie sheet. Bake at 225 degrees for 1 hour and 15 minutes..

Per serving (excluding unknown items): 50.7 Calories; 4.8 Fat (80.9 calories from fat); 1.1 Protein; 1.4 Carbohydrate; 0 Cholesterol; 9 Sodium.

Index